DOSE

Personal Prescriptions for a Happier Life and 52 Science Based Ways to Get it

Kelly

I hope you find a DOSE of happiness within...!

Julia
:)

POWERED BY

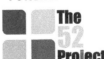

The 52 Project

Cani

Top Right Thinking Ltd
www.toprightthinking.com
Cygnet Park, 4 Office Village, Forder Way,
Hampton, Peterborough, PE7 8GX

First published in Great Britain 2023.
Copyright © Dulcie Shepherd Swanston and Iain Price, PhD.

Designed and typeset by Noodle Juice Ltd.

ISBN: 978-1-916-0853-9-8
1 3 5 7 9 10 8 6 4 2

Dedication

For Jamie, Lyra, Amelie, and Amelia – my lockdown tribe.

Dulcie

For Daniel, Joseph, Anna and Lisa - my wonderful crew; for my sister Karen and lastly for Wilki whose example and legacy lives on.

Iain

Lockdown made the gap between those who have homes and support networks, and those who do not, impossible to ignore. We want to dedicate this book to everyone who helps people who are homeless to re-build their lives, especially our friends at the Big Issue Foundation.

And for Jen. Without your technical brilliance and your dedication to The52Project not only would it not have got off the ground, but it wouldn't have stayed on the tracks either! You are amazing.

About the authors

Dulcie Shepherd Swanston

Is the owner of Profitably Engaged, Top Right Thinking and Tea Break Training which between them cover her various business strands including Executive Coaching, Public Speaking, Bite-size Training and running programmes that qualify people to become professionally accredited executive coaches and business mentors. She is also an Associate Director at People Untapped.

She previously spent over 20 years in leadership roles across Brand Development, Commercial, Operations and Human Resources for a FTSE 250 company.

Her work has been cited in diverse publications from the *Sunday Telegraph* to *The Sun* and she has featured on BBC 5 Live and BBC online. She believes herself to be the only Fellow of the CIPD who also has an MBA and a qualification as a nightclub bouncer.

Dulcie had an ironic and unhelpful limiting belief prior to lockdown that she would not enjoy or be capable of operating the technology that would enable her to coach and train to virtual audiences. Post lockdown she has had to eat her words and now works with leaders across the world and has added Starbucks, GSK, Amcor and Swiss Re to the clients she is proud to support in hospitality, retail, technology and communications.

She lives between Warwickshire and the seaside at Tynemouth with her husband, two dogs and between one and five of their older children. She is foolish enough to have taken #Tip1 to extremes and can now be found in the North Sea without a wet suit - in winter.

Find out more about Top Right Thinking at:
www.toprightthinking.com
Find out more about Dulcie at:
www.linkedin.com/in/dulcieshepherd

Iain Price, PhD

Is the founding director of Think it Out: an associate community of coaches, trainers, facilitators, authors, speakers and consultants who help people by unlocking, releasing, elevating and inspiring creative and connected thinking. Not only does this open possibility and opportunity for their clients it is also intentionally a collaborative platform for much needed positive social and environmental initiatives.

Iain studied neuroscience at university, going on to gain his doctorate in how neural cells decide what to be when grown in flasks (like petri dishes) then working as a research scientist in academic, biotech and hospital settings. He loved the creative and collaborative aspects of doing science but found lab work limited his opportunity for interaction and wider conversation with people (Iain talked a grown man to tears aged 3). Leaving the lab, he completed a postgraduate diploma in science communication. He was the neuroscientist for the BBC's *Human Mind* community outreach programmes before working for two UK charities that continue to raise confidence in students and teachers through effective communication and mindset workshops.

Iain evolved his communication skills gaining an executive coaching qualification. He now coaches, trains, facilitates and speaks using applied theory and psychometrics to help individuals, organisations, companies, not-for-profits and charities to lead through change. He challenges and connects their thinking helping them to untap, unleash and realise – to grow – possibilities together: to 'think it out'. In short, to be more together.

Find out more about Think it Out at:
www.thinkitout.co.uk
Find out more about Iain at:
www.linkedin.com/in/driainprice

Contents

Introduction

The Big Idea

I (Dulcie) remember the exact moment I had the idea for what became The 52 Project. It was a December night in 2020. The Christmas tree was up and twinkling, the fire was blazing. We were enjoying a glass of wine on a Saturday night with four of our five teenagers actually in the room with us. I had one of those moments when you feel really contented.

I have trained my brain to notice, pause and actively narrate when I am feeling positive because I know about the scientific power of 'gratitude journalling' (see #Tip3). I do all of this in my own mind – without comment of course, as I fully appreciate that the teenagers would leave the room and the moment would be lost!

At that moment I would have told myself something like, "I'm noticing this feels lovely. I am so grateful to have a lovely and warm home and for the fact that in this moment, we are a family enjoying simply being in a room together."

I don't do this gratitude journalling naturally. It is one of a number of learnt behaviours I actively practise to stay mentally well – that I have 'wired in'. I suffered from depression a little while ago and was on medication for two years and I really wanted to find other ways to improve and support my mental health so that I could help myself to stay well without necessarily having long term medication.

When I wasn't well and started to investigate proven ways that could bolster up my mental fitness, I already knew myself well. I discarded anything complicated, or that I would find boring. I was time poor and low on energy, so quick and simple was the order of the day. Anything that was unrealistic to commit to also went so that I didn't feel guilty about wasting money or messing people around. For example, I knew I would enjoy a regular dance class, and the science supported it, but with family and work commitments, I knew I would find it difficult to commit to an evening routine out of home – and to try would only add to the stress and frustration I was already feeling.

I also discarded anything where upon closer scrutiny, the science wasn't that strong. I really wanted to make sure that even if I was investing five minutes, it was five minutes that was definitely going to make a difference – my internal version of ROI (return on investment) I guess!

I had been taking a cold shower since January of that year. For much longer, I had been drinking a glass of beetroot juice most mornings before a walk. When I went out for the walk, I would remind myself to look at colour and shape contrasts in nature and not just catch up on phone messages.

These small things became part of my daily routine that I found myself doing without thinking, and they made a difference to me. A University College London study in 2010 reported that if you persist with something for 66 days on average, it is likely to become habitual. This had become the case with me – I had persisted with these habits for almost a year in the case of the cold showers and much longer in the case of the beetroot juice and the colour/shape watching.

Cast your mind back to that December night in 2020. Most of us had Christmas plans blown out of the water at the last minute. Many of us were facing Christmas without loved ones. I reflected on how grateful I was that I had discovered the science about how to deliberately increase your resilience and mood through simple daily habits before lockdown.

I started to imagine what would have happened to my mental health during 2020, if I had not had habits that were done deliberately to boost my levels of Dopamine, Oxytocin, Serotonin and Endorphins and 'wire in' habits that lifted me every day. I would not have been in a good place at all… and with that thought my brain was off!

I wondered how many people don't realise it is easy to boost positive chemicals in your brain – that in effect, doing something simple makes your body release the chemicals almost automatically. It's probably a bit unusual after all, to know that thinking grateful thoughts can boost both the affirming feeling and reward brain chemicals (neurotransmitters) serotonin and dopamine.

I started wondering how I could find an easy way to share some of the simple tips I had found to increase the levels of these chemical messengers and improved brain wiring to help people with a challenging New Year with more COVID-19 restrictions. Maybe one tip per week so it was digestible? I had an idea that I wanted a way to make science knowledge useful and accessible to my friends, family and clients – even if another year of lockdown meant I wasn't seeing them very much.

The idea of The 52 Project was born!

I had seen visuals on the internet about the acronym:

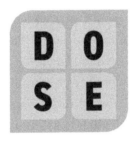

I thought that sharing tips that were scientifically shown to increase levels of the DOSE chemicals could be a great place to start.

I then thought about using Instagram Live. I'd done one for a client and found it remarkably straightforward to use the tech! Next came the idea that if I got cracking, I could launch this on the first week in January and do a tip every week for a year.

This was all happening solo in my brain on that same December night! I decided to do a bit of my pondering aloud at that stage (to use the power of many brains). I asked my family for help.

Thanks to a bit of family brainstorming, The 52 Project

was born. We found The52Project.com was available and that @the52tips was free on Instagram (someone else had got to the 'Project' option first!).

I could only think of one small problem as I went to bed. I didn't yet know 52 tips. I did a quick count and reckoned I had 20. With every problem comes an opportunity – who did I know who could add tips? And how many would come on the project as a guest?

Overnight I had a brainwave (they do happen in science!). Dr Iain Price, a neuroscientist who I had met through my work as an associate at People Untapped, was an ideal guest – but he would be an even better co-presenter with all that science literally in his head…

The only problem was I didn't know Dr Iain very well. Apart from seeing each other in a Zoom conference, we'd met for a virtual cuppa once. Given the only thing standing in the way of a great idea was calling a virtual stranger, telling him I'd had a random idea on Saturday night that I wanted to put into practice in a fortnight that required him to do something weekly that was not for profit, I decided to apply the motto from my favourite mug. It says, '*Shy Bairns Get Nowt*'.

I messaged Dr Iain and asked. He loved the idea and, having worked through depression and anxiety in the past himself, added many more of his own tips to the list. The only remaining question was, "How do we get a website up and running in less than a fortnight?" Well it turns out that wasn't so hard either. I called Digital Jen who ran my website to find out how long it would take to set up a new one and if she knew any not-for-profit organisations who do this kind of work. She pulled out all of the stops, herself, for free because she loved the idea of the project too, and by the start of January we were off!

In that moment both myself and Dr Iain were jointly setting ourselves the challenge of seeing if we could do this project, whatever it was it would become, for a whole year.

We did an Instagram Live together every Friday morning at 10am in 2021, sharing one tip every week, over a cup of tea (or water) that fulfilled five criteria. We wanted to find 52 tips that were easy to do, accessible for anyone, cheap or free, stackable with other tips – and last but not least, have credible scientific back-up, to make them fully fledged #Tips.

Digital Jen went from, "I better turn up to a 'Live' to be supportive [of my clients]," to one of our most enthusiastic testers (experimenters) of the #Tips, adding a lot more ideas and support to the project along the whole way, even co-presenting many Lives with us. We had at least already one convert!

The 52 Project moved quickly from being a solo lockdown idea into a wonderful community-styled science project where friends, family and complete strangers came together and explored everything – well-being tips that were famous old wives' tales and niche items from the Internet or science journals, to, "I've just done this thing, it sounds a bit strange but…" Each week looked into which #Tips had real scientific legs and which were snake oil. We asked our testers to try them in real life and to give us their #Tips about how to make them stick for real people in the real world. To find which were worth five minutes of your time and which weren't. This book is a summary and celebration of everything we found out together as a community. It turns out that I needn't have worried about knowing 52 tips myself, our community of people who joined us either live or recorded, had plenty for us to investigate! Together we learnt so much from each other and through the experience, that it has literally become part of our lives and daily positive well-being habits for life.

To make this book easier to navigate, and quick to read, each chapter has a #Tip in summary – *The Big Idea*

Some people might want to know more about **What's the Science?** – so that is the next section.

We then give you some *Stack Suggestions* – #Tips that are related or work well together so you can get an extra bang for your buck! To check out the science references and other further resources, including the original Instagram Live recordings, for each #Tip, head to our website: https://the52project.com.

We finish each #Tip by sharing some of the learning and reflections from our community – either *Tales from our Testers* or *Parting Shots* – something we learnt as a community from real life that helped us to make a #Tip stick – maybe an adaptation that made it easier or more flexible. We also highlight some of the key neurochemicals (**DOSE**) that scientists believe to be in play by doing these #Tips.

You don't need to read each chapter or #Tip in order, each is meant to be self-contained with all that you need to start using it in one place. Of course, the more you read and try the different #Tips, the more you are likely to get familiar with the underlying concepts which should give you greater mastery of your own well-being #Tips and habits. This is so important, because so much of what we all do day-to-day is habitual – what we end up doing without consciously (being aware of) thinking about. If you are coming at this book with some specific concerns, or especially feeling low or unconfident in certain ways, we have set out some recommendations next to help get you started too.

So what are you waiting for? We invite you to read on for 52 Tips, so that you can form your own personal prescriptions (habits) to feel happier, live well or just get an energy or mood boost, as and when you might need.

Prepare Your Personal Prescriptions

We are aware there a lot of #Tips and a lot of information in your hands right now which can make it difficult to know where to start.

When we started The52Project, we were not sure if we could do it; to come up with 52 low to no cost #Tips that would be accessible to almost everyone and anyone. They needed to have little demand on the pressures and restrictions of national lockdowns, which would also translate to elevate time-strapped busy lives post-lockdowns. Like so many habits, it was a matter of stepping into the adventure together, one step at a time, whilst believing in the premise that we could (#Tip**45**), and that we would find what we needed to find, and who to connect with (#Tip**34**), in and through the process of doing it. One of our favourite quotes is from Aristotle, used by Albert Einstein, "for the things we have to learn before doing them, we learn by doing them". We believe this can be for you too, despite how you might be feeling to the contrary right now. Why? Because we witnessed and felt the impact with family, friends, fellow '52 experimenters' and contributors, associates, colleagues and clients – people like you – each and every day.

The heart of The52Project is to provide practical and useful #Tips to make a difference in your life, wherever you are, however you might be feeling. So we have put some suggested #Tips for you to try in answer to some of the bigger questions we and our testers faced. These are only suggestions. We strongly encourage you to explore others as you get some great #Tips, that become habits and part of your daily routines, under your belt. Remember, one of the keys to success here is to 'habit stack' (put together or layer) the #Tips. Use the questions and suggestions below and on the next pages as the springboard to learn what you need to learn, to have more of the happier life that you want, need and deserve. These are set out as suggested #Tips with complementary 'stacks'. The main thing is, to have something different or more worthwhile, you need to start somewhere. If you are still struggling to know where to start, see #Tip**45**.

So, in no particular order – and do allow yourself to pick and mix, mix and match – try some of these questions to help spark and start your own 52 journey:

Struggling with change?				Want more daily energy levels?		
Try from		Stack with		Try from		Stack with
#Tip **13** #Tip **27** #Tip **35**		#Tip **21** #Tip **28** #Tip **45**		#Tip **4** #Tip **24** #Tip **29**		#Tip **7** #Tip **17** #Tip **33**

Do you need some motivation and inspiration?				Are you after a quick energy boost?		
Try from		Stack with		Try from		Stack with
#Tip **9** #Tip **11** #Tip **23**		#Tip **12** #Tip **38** #Tip **40** #Tip **50**		#Tip **1** #Tip **4** #Tip **14**		#Tip **7** #Tip **16** #Tip **43**

Do you need more head space and time to think?

Try from

#Tip #Tip #Tip
2 **3** **48**

Stack with

#Tip #Tip #Tip
13 **27** **49**

Need some focus in your life?

Try from

#Tip #Tip #Tip
9 **19** **35**

Stack with

#Tip #Tip #Tip
7 **28** **31**

Feeling overwhelmed, low or fragile?

Try from

#Tip #Tip #Tip #Tip
2 **5** **21** **47**

Stack with

#Tip #Tip #Tip #Tip
13 **15** **31** **39**

Worried you are missing out on life?

Try from

#Tip #Tip #Tip
3 **9** **35**

Stack with

#Tip #Tip #Tip
26 **34** **37**

Need help with sleep?

Try from

#Tip #Tip #Tip
24 **33** **39**

Stack with

#Tip #Tip #Tip
11 **15** **21**

Struggling with the season?

Try from

4 **11** **24**

Stack with

6 **30** **41**

Want more challenge or excitement in your life?

Try from

#Tip #Tip #Tip #Tip
23 **26** **34** **43**

Stack with

#Tip #Tip #Tip #Tip
8 **27** **32** **45**

Feeling short of time to do something that can make a positive difference for you?

Try from

#Tip #Tip #Tip
27 **28** **35**

Stack with

7 **5** **16**

Feeling lonely or struggling to connect?

Try from

18 **25** **34**

Stack with

#Tip #Tip #Tip
21 **26** **36**

Are you holding onto stress, tension or hurt?

Try from

#Tip #Tip #Tip #Tip
13 **28** **31** **39**

Stack with

#Tip #Tip #Tip
2 **21** **46**

Want to know how nutrition can legally turbo charge your thinking, resilience and recovery?

Try from

#Tip #Tip #Tip
7 **14** **31**

Stack with

#Tip #Tip #Tip
5 **41** **46**

Want to feel generally healthier?

Try from   Stack with

Do you get stuck or incapacitated by fear or shyness?

Try from   Stack with

Want to know how to help others?

Try from   Stack with

Want to get better concentration?

Try from   Stack with

Want some #Tips to do with your children?

Try from   Stack with

 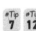

Are you dealing with failure or bereavement?

Try from   Stack with

Need some #Tips you can do (almost) anywhere, anytime?

Try from   Stack with

Do you feel lost, at a loss or lonely?

Try from   Stack with

Want to know how to make habits stick better?

Try from   Stack with

Want something to awaken and tantalise your senses?

Try from   Stack with

Want to feel more in control of life?

Try from

Stack with

Need more patience or struggling to see the future could be positive?

Try from

Stack with

Want to feel like you can and have more confidence in your abilities?

Try from

Stack with

Want to increase your options and chances of success and happiness?

Try from

Stack with

Do you want to be more?

Try from

Stack with

Do you need to be more productive or efficient (do more)?

Try from

Stack with

Want greater success and fulfilment in your relationships?

Try from

Stack with

Do you need greater resilience (and are prepared to work at it)?

Try from

Stack with

Do you feel totally overwhelmed or desperate?

Do reach out to your doctors and you could connect with these people:

Mind

www.mind.org.uk /
@mindcharity (Twitter
& Instagram) /
mindforbettermentalhealth
(Facebook)

The Samaritans

www.samaritans.org /
@samaritanscharity
(Instagram & Facebook) /
@Samaritans (Twitter)

Alcoholics Anonymous

www.aa.org & https://www.
alcoholics-anonymous.org.uk /
@aa_12steps (Instagram)

Christians Against Poverty (CAP)

https://capuk.org /
capuk_org (Instagram) /
@CAPuk (Twitter & Facebook)

Step Change (Debt Charity)

www.stepchange.org /
@StepChange (Twitter) /
@stepchangedebtcharity
(Facebook)

Professional Accredited Counselling & Therapy Finder (do check therapists' accreditations & qualifications)

www.bacp.co.uk (UK),
www.aapweb.com (USA),
www.pacfa.org.au (Australia),
https://nzac.org.nz
(New Zealand),
www.therapist-directory.co.za
(South Africa),
www.therapyroute.com
(International)

#Tip
1 Cold Showers

The Big Idea

At the end of your normal hot shower, you turn the dial and make it cold for the last 30 seconds. A quick blast of freezing cold water jolts your body and mind, which science suggests, might be really good for us for all sorts of reasons – some we don't even understand properly yet.

This is such a simple hack – quick, easy and you are done and dusted in 30 seconds … what's not to like?

Well quite a lot according to our feedback!

Imagine you are having a lovely warm shower. Maybe you can see out of the window into your frosty garden. The steam is rising. You are warm and relaxed…

Imagine how hard it is to take the simple step of turning the dial so that your shower is suddenly freezing cold. We've done it … and trust us… It was really, really hard to turn that dial!

Got it... What's the Science?

When something is hard to do because it doesn't feel like it is going to bring us pleasure, our brains give us plenty of excuses to put it off until tomorrow. Certainly, in our experience, it is still tempting to skip a day when it's a dark

morning and there is a cold wind blowing outside!

Firstly, it appears that the sudden cold shock gives us an endorphin rush as a reward, a way to take the edge off. Most of our 'willing' testers of #Tip1 said they felt fantastic afterwards. Whilst this could just be connected to the temperature of the water, most of them reported that they felt proud of themselves for being brave enough to try it.

After doing vigorous exercise our bodies can release endorphins. These are our 'coping' biochemicals and hormones. Endorphins are also the body's natural opioid like pain killers and they can make us feel good. So, challenging our bodies with cold can give us a pleasurable endorphin hit.

Secondly, there is an evolutionary premise that we have a 'calling' or 'harking' back to the sea and cold water. This is part of Edward O. Wilson's 'biophilia' hypothesis, where connection with nature is 'ingrained' in our genes (see #Tip11). For the ocean, Wallace J. Nichols terms this ancestorial-to-present connection the 'Blue Mind'. Our ancient ancestors would have seen immersion in cold water as a positive thing. It appears that whilst the cold water might take our breath away initially, it can act to slow our breathing and heart rate down through the 'mammalian diving reflex'. This reflex is complicated, but suffice it to say, for our purposes, that it is a protective and multifaceted physiological reaction that prepares our bodies for immersion and can even be trance-like. It might be that whilst our conscious modern brains go, "Wow, no way, you must be joking?" to the idea of a cold shower, part of more primal brain architecture welcomes the cold water – and, as a result, at some deeper level, it feels really good.

Cold water therapy is an ancient Ayurvedic (Sanskrit words *ayur* for life; and *veda* for science or knowledge) remedy for anxiety and depression, now backed by modern science. A study at the Virginia Commonwealth University found that cold showers can alleviate and may even prevent anxiety and depression. The author Nikolai Shevchuk claims that the short cold showers stimulate the 'blue-spot' (*Locus Coeruleus*) in the brain, a primary place for producing noradrenaline (a neurotransmitter), which could help with depression and anxiety.

A BBC TV show with Hugh Fearnley-Whittingstall showed Hugh experiencing cold water swimming in a bid to reduce his own anxiety and depression. This programme was backed by scientists who suggested that the benefits may arise because being immersed in cold water is a stress trigger. When the body experiences stress by a physical 'hostile' external factor – in this case cold water – a coping response in the body is stimulated in the body to 'cope' with and 'repair' the 'damage' caused by the hostile factor. In the case of the 30 second cold shower, there is no real 'threat', but our body and brain don't know that. It gives us all the benefits that it would if the threat was a real and present danger – rather than a slightly shocking, but probably not at all dangerous, pastime which only lasts 30 seconds!

Finally, our testers suggested that regular cold showering makes them feel ready for battle and that smaller things that might make them ordinarily quite reactive – maybe make them cry or get angry – didn't seem to bother them as much on cold shower days. However, it seems probable that our 'fight or flight' mechanisms are triggered by the cold-water shock – certainly in our experience it is something you want to fight doing or get out of as quickly once that 30 seconds is over! Given this is the case, it may be that this physical and quite brutal cold shock 'desensitises' some of our 'fight or flight'. So things that would ordinarily get our heckles up, are put more into perspective. We perceive them as less challenging or more manageable.

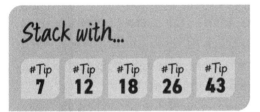

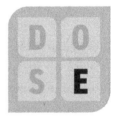

Tales from our Testers

"Okay, so after much protestation I just did the cold shower thing and whilst it wasn't very pleasant I will reluctantly admit I'm feeling quite smug and good right now."

Helen Melvin, People Director, Brasserie Bar Co, Twickenham, England

#Tip 2 Warm Afternoon Bath

The Big Idea

OK, so this one is really easy to sell! At least twice a week, take a hot bath in the afternoon for 30 minutes. Ideally, follow it by another 20 minutes taking it easy and staying warm. We appreciate that #Tip1 'Cold Showers', might have taken a bit of courage or be something you needed to work up to, so here is a brain boosting tip that is a bit easier to imagine yourself getting into!

Taking regular afternoon baths has been shown to have a positive and measurable lift in mood for people suffering from mild to moderate depression. In fact, those people involved in the study found that hot baths could be even more effective than physical exercise as a mood booster.

Got it... What's the Science?

Researchers from the University of Freiburg in Germany studied a group of 36 people who were experiencing depression. About half of them were on medication and continued with it during the trial. The participants were split randomly into two groups. Half started going to a spa for a soak twice per week and the other group did supervised

exercise twice per week. Researchers studied them to see which activity seemed to help most with their mood.

After just two weeks of hot baths, the people in that group reported a positive impact on their mood. The group who did the exercise did experience a mood lift, but it took longer to experience the uplift. Giving a quicker return might have also meant that few people dropped out of the hot bath group.

After eight weeks of hot baths, participants reported a 6-point improvement in their mood. Those doing the exercise did report an improvement, but by 3 points.

The study wasn't huge or perfect, in fact the comparison group who were doing the physical exercise had more people drop out – which might suggest that a hot bath habit is easier for more people to keep up than an exercise one.

The reason it works is believed to involve our circadian rhythms and body clock. These are, and set, the daily routines of biological processes that synchronise our daily functioning and well-being. In a nutshell, our bodies get into rhythms and cycles so that we excrete the right biochemicals to co-ordinate processes and behaviours to match the relevant time of the day. You will experience this as feeling hungry at regular mealtimes and feeling alert or sleepier at certain times of day.

Our core body temperature usually rises during the daytime, peaking in the late afternoon and falling overnight. This temperature cycle is a cue to your body clock. However, when people experience depression, this temperature cycle is often flatter or delayed by several hours – so the temperature peak comes at a less appropriate time which can affect body functions like sleep.

The afternoon bath can comfortingly simulate and 'mark' the body temperature peak to match a healthier daily rhythm. This helps the body to know what time, or part of the daily routine, it is. In theory this should apply for everyone. Although the study was small, the science around circadian rhythms means that the findings make sense. Douglas Adams, author of *The Hitch-hikers Guide to the Galaxy*, was a famous afternoon bath fan.

Other studies have shown that taking a warm bath before bed can also help you to sleep providing you have a cool room to sleep in afterwards (about 18 to 20°C is ideal). Poor sleep is associated with most mental health and well-being issues. So, another reason that warm baths might help reduce depression is that they help people to sleep better by giving a more defined temperature gradient or 'step' (differential) before going to sleep.

There could be another reason why it seems to work ... a hot bath just feels lovely! For an extra mood boost try adding some lavender or ylang-ylang oil to your bath – we'll also look at aromatherapy and scents in #Tip15!

If you are lucky enough to have access to a hot tub, then definitely jump in! Hot tubs can be more easily shared and this social aspect is known to be beneficial, so you could have a double dose of well-being boost sharing a hot tub. If you can do this outside, you could also get the combined benefit of sunlight, vitamin-D or a spot of mindful nature watching.

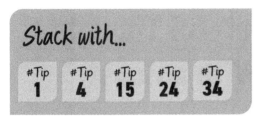

Stack with...

#Tip **1** #Tip **4** #Tip **15** #Tip **24** #Tip **34**

Parting Shot

Unless you are suffering from a heart condition, which makes it dangerous to experience any sudden change in temperature, this one seems to be worth a two-week trial.

The water needs to be pretty hot – the study we mention here used water at 40°C. If you don't have a thermometer, don't worry, 40°C is not super-extreme. It will feel hot when you get in – but it's not scalding or too uncomfortable.

#Tip 3 Grateful Thoughts – With a Boost

The Big Idea

Write them down! The simple process of reflecting on and writing down things that you are grateful for releases feel good hormones and transmitters in your brain (serotonin (also called 5-hydroxytryptamine or 5-HT) and dopamine) which in turn helps you train – 'wire' – your brain to see the positive opportunities and aspects in people and life. In her book, *It's Not Bloody Rocket Science*, Dulcie speaks of a Native American parable of feeding two wolves that battle within us: positivity or negativity. When you choose to feed the positive (grateful) wolf you are cultivating that part of your thinking and growing that part of your personality.

Most of us have an internal voice. If you recognise this phenomenon, this voice is the person you live with 24/7. Choosing which voice to cultivate and listen to will ultimately determine your reality.

To live happier, healthier and more successful lives we need to take control of our brain's attentional focus. Acknowledging and recognising the positives is how we begin to steer our own ship with the rudder of our attention; controlling what we focus on and so what we get.

This reminds us of the Buddha's quote: "we are what we

think" and Zig Ziglar's quote: "it is your attitude, more than your aptitude, that will determine your altitude."

The simplest and most effective way of doing this is to give yourself a few minutes each day to write down what and who you are grateful for, for that day, that week, in life generally; what compliments you would like to give yourself and what you are learning in the challenges you are facing. Go on, have a go!

Got it... What's the Science?

Part of the role of your brain and your inner voice, is to keep you safe. For the vast majority of us the internal voice can spot what could be a threat, what we have done wrong or how others could wrong us.

"So, what's the problem?" you ask. The problem is, as Tony Robins says, where your attention goes, the energy flows (or where the energy flows, the attention goes – both ways round hold up). When you focus on problems and what's wrong and allow yourself to do so by not challenging your inner voice, you get more problems and you 'see' and notice more of what's wrong in the world. This creates a perception shift caused by a brain short cut, a bias, called 'confirmation bias'.

This is where the Reticular Activating System (RAS) comes in. Part of its job is to allow us to filter out unnecessary information and alert us to when something is important. So, if we are not careful, it will be on constant alert to what could be wrong – rather than what could be right.

Lack of awareness or inability to use this brain science is one of our main restrictors, holding back our progress. Conversely, effective people and entrepreneurs such as Elon Musk and Richard Branson are so successful because their brains have instead been 'wired' and tuned through repeated practice to notice opportunities that bring them, and their teams, success and fulfilment.

It is well known that the roots of many psychopathological conditions such as acute anxiety and stress, even chronic pain, are not just related to, but caused by, unhappiness.

Researchers and meditative practitioners, such as Emily Fletcher – founder of Ziva, have referred to gratitude as a natural anti-depressant, where the impact of practising gratitude daily, like keeping a gratitude journal, can be similar to anti-depressant medications.

This is because the process of just thinking and processing and, even better, sharing gratitude, releases serotonin and dopamine, two key neurotransmitters in the regulation of our emotions. Their release generally makes us feel good. Also, your brain seeks out opportunities for releasing these hormones as a reward for what makes us feel better. So, the more frequently you are grateful, the more likely you are to notice opportunities to be grateful for. It's a positive feedback loop.

Put this together with your RAS and you have a powerful way of feeling better and orientating 'automatically' to opportunities that are going to bring you more happiness and most likely success. You are also more likely to spot positives in people around you and help them to see them for themselves as well. These are the kind of people most of us would want to be around and trust, so you and your brain can become your own mutual best friends and cheer leaders.

And the benefits don't just stop there! A raised level of gratitude is known to be associated with a reduction in stress hormones such as cortisol, associated with heart disease; a reduced subjective perception of pain; an improved likelihood of refreshing and energising sleep; an improved ability to deal with stress and a release from toxic emotions and memories that hold us back as well as improving social cohesion with more fulfilled, healthier support interconnections with those that matter most to us.

ALL this from just a bit of gratitude! What are you waiting for?

D O
S E

Parting Shot

If you prefer, instead of writing you could doodle your thoughts or even audio record them. It is the process of processing your gratitude (i.e. thinking it out) that is most important here. This could be the beginning of a journalling habit so maybe treat yourself to a new journal so you can dedicate some clear and private thinking space. Maybe even enjoy a cuppa while you gather your thoughts.

4 Morning Sunshine

The Big Idea

We know that we are solar powered. What do we mean? We mean we work best when we both have had regular access to sunshine – ideally with fresh, clean air. This doesn't have to be warm, just bright light.

It has been known since ancient times that sunlight can have a big impact on our sense of well-being and can even be therapeutic, although too much can also be damaging. Moderate exposure to early morning sunlight seems to have the most benefit for our mood, sleep and a sense of well-being.

Got it... What's the Science?

Our brains are incredibly well designed for visual processing and our eyes, although not as sensitive as other animals', are very receptive to light. We have a relatively small nucleus of multiple 'circadian oscillator' ('day cycle') neurons behind our eyes at the cross-over of optic nerves that together are called the Suprachiasmatic Nucleus (SCN). This SCN is our master circadian (day) clock, whose cells are very sensitive to light levels – even when our eyes are closed. These cells set our daily body-clock and day-night / wake-sleep rhythm. See also #Tip2.

Light, via the optic nerves running from our eyes, literally stimulates our brain and leads to activity in lots of different parts of our brain – in fact much of the back of the head parts of our brain are involved in visual processing.

But that's not the only part of our body that is light sensitive. Our skin is also receptive to sunlight, allowing us to make vitamin-D, which keep bones, teeth and muscles healthy. UV-light exposure to our skin is also linked with release of nitric oxide which is known to be beneficial to our blood pressure and cardiovascular system.

So taken together we are very light sensitive and light receptive creatures.

Season Affected Disorder (SAD) is a type of depression that many of us experience recurrently at certain times of the year, most notably the winter months in further northern or southern latitudes. Depression is a low mood which lasts over an extended period of time. Symptoms of SAD include: lack of energy, difficulty in concentrating, not wanting to be with people, sleep issues, lower libido, feelings of despair and / or changes in appetite and eating.

Like so many disorders, SAD is at one end of a spectrum or continuum of 'normal' health. So even if you don't clinically suffer SAD, it is very common to experience mild 'symptoms' when the days are dark and the nights are long.

The good news is research by medics and scientists suggest that only moderate amounts of sunlight are needed to ward off the negative impacts a lack of sunlight can have. It is known that those that work outside, especially also in winter, are much less likely to suffer from SAD or SAD-like symptoms. Plus, widely available artificial daylight bulbs (those that have a higher blue wavelength light component than normal electric bulbs) can be used to provide a cost-effective way of giving those brains that live more in the dark, access to their fix of sunlight. These are sometimes called light boxes or SAD lamps. As little as 15–20 minutes of daily bright, real or such artificial daylight can ward off the negative impacts that the lack of light can cause.

The science doesn't stop there! We know that light exposure is also associated with the release of serotonin in your brain – the often quoted 'happy hormone' and neurotransmitter. So, there are number of direct links between (sun)light, our brains and happiness.

The use of artificial daylight bulbs has also been shown to significantly improve the health and well-being of dementia patients – including improving their concentration.

Still not convinced about the benefits of sunlight? Research looking at hospital stays over 15 years, have shown that hospital stays are proportionally lower in patients who were staying closer to a window. Even more than this, some mental health patients on the east (sunrise facing) side of a hospital are likely to recover more quickly and be discharged quicker than those on the westerly side of a hospital (sunset facing).

These are many examples of how exposure to sunlight, especially at earlier parts of our waking hours, helps us feel more in sync with the day and ourselves, raising our sense of well-being and even improving our ability to concentrate.

So, this week's top tip is to try and take time to get at

least 15 minutes daylight each morning. Maybe 'habit stack' with #Tip**5** and some deliberate, mindful breathing.

Parting Shot

Too much sunlight and UV exposure is known to be linked with skin cancers, so please show restraint and sensibly use a sunscreen / sunblock on your skin (consider your skin type and consult a health professional if in any doubt) and always avoid looking directly at the sun (even with sunglasses on). We also strongly discourage the use of UV beds or lights.

Always check that daylight bulbs and light boxes are UV protected / filtered – this should be certified on the product. Also, try and avoid blue light as much as possible as it comes to bedtime.

And Breathe

The Big Idea

We all breathe but do we do it well? This might sound like a silly question but talking with Cathy Hart, vocal coach extraordinaire, we found out that a truly life changing tip is as simple as a quick morning breathing exercise to set us up for the day.

The bottom line is we can all get in our own way in 'doing', and breathing is definitely one of those things. Most of us could, it turns out, actually do with using our conscious thinking brain, Pre-Frontal Cortex (PFC), to deliberately let go and allow our body to do what it does best.

Cathy's top tip is spending at least a minute connecting with your breath before you get out of bed in the morning, to consciously 'check in' and listen to how our body is actually preferring to breathe.

Lie on your back and allow the bed to take the weight of your body. If you feel an arch in your back with your legs stretched out, lift your knees so that your feet are flat on the bed. Take a breath in through your nose and relax as you let it out gently. Just let your body breathe without interference. Doing this first thing after waking, means it should be easier to get back to the type of breathing you were doing whilst asleep. Which, when not snoring, is the most unconscious or 'natural' breathing you can do.

Next, heighten your awareness to the breath moving in and out of your body. Feel how relaxed and balanced your body feels, how free and flexible your ribs and surrounding muscles. If you feel any tension in your body, mentally let go of it and continue allowing the breath to move unrestricted in and out of your body. Where do you feel the breath? Are your chest and shoulders now relatively still? Can you feel your tummy rise up towards the ceiling when you breathe in and gently fall to the bed when breathing out? Allow the breath in and out through your nose and then in and out through your mouth – notice how your breathing changes. Ideally spending at least a minute doing this each morning allows you to tune into your own more 'natural' unforced breathing pattern.

Got it... What's the Science?

As humans, we can carry a lot of tension in our bodies as and when we're up and about. This interferes with our muscular and skeletal balance, and the resulting imbalance negatively impacts our breathing. Bad posture, tight abdominals, stress, anxiety – all these things can affect our body's natural balance and breathing.

We breathe around 25,000 times a day, and the way we breathe can help to fuel and heal our bodies if done properly. Breathing is our main source of life, feeding our cells – you can do without food for weeks; water for hours if not days, but we all need air (oxygen) and most can't do without it for four minutes or less without starting to incur brain damage. Breathing is also one of our main ways of expelling metabolic waste, namely carbon dioxide, from our body.

Fast or slow breathing? There is a big difference in the impact on your body.

Fast breathing at rest is often shallow and is associated with panic breathing and distress. Rapid breathing means that only about 25% of the air going into the lungs is actually being used. Slow breathing on the other hand means about 85% of air is actually used. Breathing slow and 'low', as in allowing air to go naturally deeper in your lungs, is far more beneficial, not only in improving our metabolism, but also in improving your body's ability to lower your blood pressure, sleep and heal itself. This is because parasympathetic nerve receptors in the lower lungs are associated with calming the mind and body, whereas the upper lung breathing can prompt hyperventilating and trigger sympathetic nerve receptors heightening the threat response of Fight, Flight, Freeze or Flock states.

Mouth or nose breathing? It matters!

Nasal (nose) breathing means air passes over the nasal mucosa which stimulate the body's reflex nerves that control the more relaxed, low breathing. Whereas, mouth breathing bypasses nasal mucosa complicating and compromising the natural reflex to breathe fully. Mouth breathing also accelerates water loss that can contribute to dehydration over the day. See also #Tip**7**. Also, we know that air passing through the nose passes over the olfactory bulbs, which is the most immediate extension of your brain – with direct access to the limbic complex involved in emotion and some important aspects of memory including the amygdala and hippocampus, as well as the hypothalamus which unconsciously controls your heart rate, blood pressure, circulation, digestion and hormone balance (see #Tip15). So, it's safe to say that nose breathing brings more than you might expect! In other words, breathing is so, so much more than just getting oxygen for metabolism into your body.

Parting Shot

Practising this exercise helps us more easily recognise when we are not breathing in this more natural way. Take a moment at any time in the day to recalibrate, back to how we felt when breathing first thing in the morning with our deliberately relaxed, low and slow breathing.

Deliberately encouraging ourselves to breathe low and slow is a truly top way of quickly calming our brains to better cope with stress, allowing us to be more in control and think more clearly and creatively to resolve problems. Breathing! Who'd have thought there was so much to it?

#Tip 6 # Do the Plank

The Big Idea

We all know how important exercise can be to wake us up, look after our blood pressure, improve our concentration and our body's ability to deal with stress. The last few years has seen an explosion in HIIT (High Intensity Interval Training) as the answer to keeping fit at home, but this easily takes up more time than the 10–15 minutes promised in adverts as the total daily time investment. Plus doing HIIT 'cold' can lead to injury. We sought out advice from gym and personal trainer guru Hedge Haigh. Cue 'strength training', which he persuaded us can give you many of the daily well-being and stress protective benefits without all the excess sweat! Yes really!

You could choose sit-ups, but this can have some down sides such as causing stress on your back's discs and doing these from cold can lead to muscle strain and back pain – not good!

Push-ups can be hard to get into and build up to if you are a complete novice. Also, not everyone wants to build up their arm strength AND push-ups can lead to some serious sweating!

So, this tip can truly help you get your quick daily exercise fix, with all the benefits and less of the faff. It's called THE PLANK! Now stay with us on this! You don't have to be 'ripped' or 'built' to do the plank – honest!

The most common plank is the forearm plank which is held in a push-up like position with the body's weight borne on forearms, elbows, and toes.

There are variations of this standard front plank, such as the side plank and the reverse plank, but for our tip we are going to just focus on the front plank version.

According to Runners World's experts, Noam Tamir, owner of TS Fitness in New York City, Danielle Zickl and Stuart McGill Ph.D., author of Ultimate Back Fitness and Performance, this is what we need to do to do a good front plank:

Ensure your elbows are on the ground directly underneath your shoulders with your feet hip-width apart. Make sure your back is flat and your head and neck are in a neutral position [that's your head not looking up or down – imagine having a broom handle that can rest flat on your head down your back]. Drive your elbows into the floor, and squeeze your quads, glutes and core (stomach muscles). Inhale through your nose and exhale through your mouth – don't hold your breath.

Research shows that for most people, holding a plank for one minute at a time creates a resilient torso but if you have a history of back pain, hold for 10 second increments to reduce your risk of back pain triggers.

Certainly, long planks are not good for you and defeat the object of having a quick tip. So just build it up, starting with smaller time targets that are still challenging for you.

Got it... What's the Science?

When you use the plank regularly to build your strength, you feel just that little bit stronger, fitter, more flexible and more confident in your own skin – a bit like putting on a confident outfit that invokes a more confident mindset. This head state tends to automatically mean we have more upright and open body postures, which as Amy Cuddy famously advocates, raises testosterone (the confidence hormone) and lowers cortisol (a stress hormone). This means you will project, and feel, more positivity internally and externally. And we know that when we feel and look more confident, other people see this and tend to react more positively to us and our ideas – which in turn makes us feel even more confident still! (This is an example of a positive feedback loop – that you can instigate.)

Core Strength and Flexibility: there are a lot of arguments as to what the core is BUT suffice to say they are the muscles that are needed to hold our stature, posture and prevent your internal organs from literally dropping out. Good core strength also helps us to have and keep good body posture during the day. We know from #Tip**5**, that body posture is also key to how we can more naturally, and healthily, breathe. Also, building core strength, especially when we are desk-bound or have a relatively sedentary lifestyle, helps prevent us from injuring ourselves when we do actually get properly active.

Muscle Tone: By holding the plank you are also stretching your muscles which stimulate nerves in these muscles and your body which, in turn, stimulate your brain and release endorphins that promote a sense of well-being. We strongly suspect that when we achieve even just this simple task routinely, there are dopaminergic rewards (from achieving body training) and serotonergic (from planning for positivity) boosts too.

Increased Metabolic Rate: it is suggested that doing a quick plank at the start and end of the day kick-starts your body to ramp up its energy use in readiness for a more active day (even if it is not so). This is particularly powerful when combined or 'stacked' with #Tip29.

Parting Shot

D O
S E

Remember to look after your back and to adapt the exercise if doing it causes you pain.

You should definitely avoid the plank, or proceed with extreme caution, if you suffer or have any of these conditions: prolapse, prolapse surgery, pelvic pain conditions, weak or poorly functioning pelvic floor muscles, recent childbirth, acute or chronic back pain, shoulder injury, or are extremely overweight.

How about seeking out a local Yoga, Pilates or gym professional to improve your strength conditioning?

#Tip 7 The Power of a Pint

The Big Idea

Each night before you go to bed, get a pint of water and put it by your bedside. This is not to drink during the night (so you might need two glasses if you sip during the night), this pint is especially and exclusively to drink first thing in the morning when you wake up. This idea is so simple, it's hard to believe it can do so much good. But before we get into the science of why, let's talk about why it's good to be prepared.

As we know, our brain finds it much easier to do something new when we link it with something we do automatically already. So, when we are trying to build new habits into our daily routine, it makes sense to 'stack' the habits – to do them at the same time or immediately before or after something that you do without thinking about it.

Waking up is a brilliant time and cue to link in a habit each day. The simple idea is that by having a pint of water by your bed, as the first thing you see when you wake up, means you will remember to drink it and re-hydrate yourself before you do anything else.

Certainly, you could try to keep hydrated using a different method, however linking it to waking up means that there is very little to get in the way of actually making it happen. Many of us will have read articles about keeping hydrated and thought, 'right, I need to drink more water,' and then promptly forgotten about it until we are thirsty – by which point you are actually already dehydrated.

Some of our testers swear by putting their morning water in a vacuum flask to keep their water cold and fresh. It may certainly keep the side of the bed looking neat! But, however you do it, just do it! Here's why…

Got it... What's the Science?

Our bodies have a neat cue to help us drink enough water – we get thirsty! But what not everyone knows is that when you are thirsty you are already dehydrated. When we become dehydrated we feel tired, lethargic and often moody(er). But there is more to it than that. Dehydration affects our ability to think.

There are numerous studies that look at the impact of dehydration on our performance and our thinking. Repeatedly scientists find that being just mildly dehydrated (2–5%) leads to significant decline in our ability to cognitively perform (think) as well as leading to long-term health consequences.

At 2% dehydrated you may not even feel thirsty, but you will already be significantly less alert, attentive and responsive, than you are on a hydrated day.

This is because thirst and even mild dehydration leads to the release of vasopressin, a prohormone (we like this as it sounds like pro-rights), from neurons in the hypothalamus, which is converted to Arginine Vasopressin (AVP). AVP in the bloodstream in turn increases blood pressure due to vasoconstriction (reduced blood vessel diameter) which can also subsequently limit the amount of blood to brain active regions. Remember, our brains are incredibly energy and resource intensive. If blood flow to a region is reduced, it limits that region's ability to function. Blood flow to brain regions is what allows scientists using imaging and scanning techniques to identify what parts of the brain are involved in certain cognitive functions. AVP also leads to the release of the stress hormone, cortisol, and the stress responses which takes blood away from the 'clever', creatively thinking part of our brain, the Pre-Frontal Cortex (PFC) – making us less clever and more stressed in the moment. Drinking water reverses this.

This is particularly important for us first thing in the morning as when sleeping, we stop drinking water. Even if you have a sip when you wake in the night, you are still using up far more than you take on, through sweating, through excreting moisture when you breathe and by making urine in your kidneys.

In short, whilst sleeping you use more water than you can take on, so it makes a lot of sense to rehydrate first thing – before you get moving and use up any more water. Perfect habit stacking timing! If you use the point of waking up and seeing the glass or flask as a cue to remember to hydrate before you get distracted, you'll be drinking water at a time of day you need it most!

Parting Shot

There is an interesting circular trap to be avoided here too. Research has shown the importance of hydration in getting healthy sleep, with the lack of sleep (and excessive daytime sleepiness) being associated with increased dehydration. It seems that hydration also most likely plays an important part of your optimal circadian rhythm function (#Tip4 and #Tip24). So, whilst having a morning pint is certainly a good start, make sure that you remember to top up at other points in the day too. This also means being more careful about your caffeine use too (#Tip33).

Looking at the other #Tips, what other habit could you most easily stack with this one to give you the best start to your days?

#Tip 8 Pay Attention

The Big Idea

A simple way to build your brainpower involves you doing hardly anything extra at all. The trick is to be more aware about what you are doing in the moment, and making small adjustments to turn the everyday 'auto-pilot' moments into opportunities for brain growth.

Trick One: when you are out and about take a moment to look at your surroundings as a photographer might do. Look at how the tallest building is silhouetted against the sky, notice how a red road sign contrasts against a blue sky or pause to notice how many different shades of green are in a patch of grass.

Trick Two: when you are going about your daily life, use your less dominant hand to do small tasks. Change the channel or open the door with your left hand instead of your right – or vice versa if you are left-handed

These tricks involve minimal additional time and very little effort to do as you are going about your daily life anyway. What is amazing is that in doing these small things you are activating and building, as well as maintaining, millions of new pathways ('wiring') in your brain.

Got it... What's the Science?

We've already mentioned, "where the attention goes, the energy flows…," and this is actually biophysically true! When you are making these small observations you are actually doing a 'mindfulness' activity.

Two things happen in pausing to pay a slightly different form of attention to an everyday task. Firstly, you are raising it up into your consciousness and so using your PFC to help you intentionally recognise what is going on and to notice what you are thinking about. Secondly, by doing this, you are sending new bioelectric energy to different parts of your brain that otherwise would not have been 'lighting up' during that activity. Doing this encourages, makes and strengthens connections between related areas in your brain that wouldn't or haven't necessarily been quite as connected with this activity until now.

We could easily underestimate the power of such a small step but here is why, in brain-power terms, it is actually not that small at all!

The adult human brain has around 100 billion neurons and 100 trillion connections. Every time you practise a new habit you are helping a different part of your brain to 'fire-up', accessing and creating MILLIONS of pathways and connections. The more you practice this and activate those pathways, the stronger the connections become making them easier and quicker to reproduce and so make a habit.

The consequences of this for us as adult human beings

are enormous. We used to think that our brains were relatively fixed from a young age. It is only relatively recently that neuroscience has helped us to understand that you can teach an old dog new tricks!

Not being conscious of what we are doing in our daily lives nor taking action to mindfully choose to do something different, doesn't mean we are being lazy – we are doing exactly what our brain wants us to do, which is to save energy. Your brain is about 2% of your body weight but requires about 20% of your daily energy needs. So your brain is an energy miser; it doesn't spend energy unless there is a real need to or a tangible perceived benefit.

Research has suggested that by the time we are adults, up to 90% of what we think, feel and do is simply recycled frameworks from our past. So, we can potentially live quite happy lives by being on auto-pilot and replicating the things we have learnt already.

However, your brain only changes and embraces new stuff when and if you challenge it to do so, when you actively do something different and persist with it, despite it feeling a bit weird or awkward to start with.

Often the fear and uncertainty of not being as good at the new stuff is what puts us off trying, which can lead to a 'fixed mindset' – we are encouraging ourselves instead to have a 'growth mindset'. This means trying new stuff that will sometimes not work the way you thought it would. You may even 'fail', but your brain (and you) continues to learn by doing anyway.

Learning a new language or how to play a musical

instrument (in fact any complex skill) all have proven and significant impacts on our brain power. But if time is short or motivation is low, it is important to know that a little bit of something newer or different today, is better than an intention to do a big thing that you put off until 'tomorrow'.

Think about living life more intentionally – notice what's going on so you can be more able, strategic and deliberate in practising new ways of learning.

So that is why even a trying a small thing leads to a million changes! And each of those changes has the potential to make incremental differences and be the start of something much, much bigger, as we explore in the next tip.

Tales from our Testers

"I started taking a photograph on the morning walk that I do in all weathers with my dog. One of the wonderful things about this tip is that over time it has become my diary. And having done it for a full year, there is an added bonus! Sometimes I get a 'this time last year' photo from my phone which reminds me of one these photographs. It gives me a wonderful, impromptu reminder of all I have to be grateful for and how much I have gotten from these tips!"

Jane Althorpe – Customer Relations Executive, St Neots, England

Time Travel

The Big Idea

So, confession time: *Back to the Future* is probably one of our favourite films of all time. Now this probably says a lot about our age. As science geeks we have been speaking about what if we could time travel and then it hit us when talking to a colleague and therapist, Mark Evans, that we already have all the equipment we need(ish) in our own brains.

This all started for us from a study back in 2014 associated with Harvard Business School (HBS) which showed that people who were given the opportunity to reflect at the end of a working day showed 20+% boost in efficacy (efficiency in performance) in subsequent weeks at work. Not only that but as HBS professor Francesca Gino says, those who reflected felt, "more confident that they can achieve things. As a result, they put more effort into what they're doing and what they learn."

As executive and performance coaches we have found that some sort of reflection at the end of the day by thinking, especially if combined with recording reflections and insights in some way – say by journalling – massively improves the success, happiness and drive of our clients in achieving their goals. This is incredibly empowering and leads to so many more well-being benefits (#Tip3).

So, what's going on? And is it all it's cracked up to be?

Got it... What's the Science?

Our brains are busy building versions of our life all the time – they are habit and pattern 'machines'. So whether you are aware of it or not, you are constantly telling yourself stories of who you are and what is important to you, which in turn impacts the patterns that make up your brain and your mind – indeed yourself. These stories form our 'frames of reference' or as Stephen Covey calls them, 'paradigms' – the metaphoric 'lenses' through which we see and experience the world.

Like any good story, our own story includes *Back to the Future*'s theme dimension: time. As humans we, along with some animals with more developed brains like dolphins and apes, have a sense of 'self' and 'physical space' in context with events or memories. These memories are fickle in themselves as our brains are busy filtering, sifting and presenting the salient (what's subjectively deemed important) information based on the paradigms and habits it is 'running' in the background all the time. This means that different people can witness the same event but have very different memories and recall of the same physical event. As fantastic as our brains are, unlike our smart phones, they are not digital multimedia recorders (in fact they are arguably better by being analogue).

This could be seen as just a problem, but it can also be used for our own good.

Therapists like Mark Evans can use this brain capacity or quirk to invite clients suffering especially from trauma to time travel: to recall, (re)reflect and more healthily (re) interpret memories (PAST) to help them heal their own minds and bodies. We can all use this approach to deliberately and consciously raise what is important to us from our own memories, so we become much more likely recognise pertinent or 'successful' life patterns in the PRESENT, which in turn shapes our better FUTURE.

Reflecting at the end of a day – time travelling BACK, using journalling or something similar, reinforces pathways or neural connections in the brain that stand out to us, as important or relevant (salient), in the PRESENT. Those experiences and actions we took, or would have preferred to take, are then practised in our brain, wiring them together more strongly (Hebb's Postulate: 'neurons that fire together wire together'). Externalising memories from the PAST allows our brain capacity to relatively filter or 'reframe' in the PRESENT, negative components into the more positive 'mission' or 'vision' you have of yourself for the FUTURE. The more we do this, the more we are training our brains to notice what's really important and to focus on these – and so we're more likely to 'get' the subject of our focus in the future. This, in turn, frees up mental bandwidth by enabling us to have more capacity to process and manipulate new 'data' / experiences / work that we are asking our brains to manage. Bottom line, combined, we can have more intent on what will happen in the FUTURE by our PRESENT processing of the PAST. The basis of this approach is a powerful tool to facilitate our clients' thinking to their own success and fulfilment.

Stack with...

#Tip	#Tip	#Tip	#Tip	#Tip
3	**11**	**19**	**22**	**23**

Parting Shot

"We do not learn from experience... we learn from reflecting on experience." John Dewey

This technique / brain ability is also often referred to as Mental Time Travel (MTT) by therapists, psychologists and psychotherapists.

There is an important distinction and caveat here in being solution or goal focused, on what we are working towards rather what we are running away from (being afraid of).

Like all our top tips the key is doing this a bit is better than not doing it all. If you just start by reflecting (time travelling) a little each week, or even once a month, that will bring you benefits. And of course, the more you can incorporate it into a daily routine (habit stack), the more it is going to give you back in terms of return on the time you invest in it.

Combine this #Tip with **#Tip8** for powerful Jedi-like boosts in 'intentional attention'. To find out how sleep is important here, check out **#Tip19** and **#Tip35**.

#Tip
10 Keep Smiling

The Big Idea

So we all know the power of a winning smile from someone else but did you know that smiling yourself can mean you are also happier, healthier, more attractive and more successful in your work? Here's the thing: the more we smile, the more this becomes true. Smiling could possibly be the simplest most impactful habit you could make. And it's so 'stackable'!

The age-old adages of 'grin and bear it' or 'just keep smiling' may have far more credit to the secret of life than we might have taken it for. In fact, this is one that genuinely needs to be taken at more than face value!

So, what's going on? And is smiling all it's cracked up to be?

Got it... What's the Science?

When we smile our brains release a cocktail of neurotransmitters that we have already spoken about as having a positive impact on our mood and well-being: dopamine and serotonin as well as endorphins – our self-made natural painkillers. These help lower anxiety and increase feelings of happiness. Right off the bat we already know that having these in our brain help improve our ability to withstand difficulties as well as physical and emotional pain. So, smiling can immediately help increase our ability to get through challenging times and help us gain more resilience.

Smiling actually requires about as many muscles as frowning – it's just that most of us tend to do more smiling than frowning – so the effort to smile is usually easier because these muscles are stronger. An authentic smile is also generally conveyed by and revealed 'through' our eyes and this is important for a number of reasons too.

Our brains are constantly and principally scanning people's eyes and mouths when they are talking. This means that our brains are keyed into reading signals that other faces are giving us. A study at Aberdeen University, Scotland, found that those who smiled and made eye contact were consistently rated higher on the attractiveness scale than those who didn't.

And most of us find a smile is contagious – in a good way. When someone smiles, most of us find it hard to resist smiling back. Smiling is likely to be an evolutionary anthropological social cue to say, "hey I am friendly and no threat to you." The more we mutually share this, the lower our blood pressures and heart rates become. This is probably to help social cohesion and allow new collaborations between new people (tribe members) who are like us (see #Tip**34**). So, simply smiling lowers the strain on our cardiovascular systems and we know that repetitively lowering this increases life expectancy.

Decreasing our threat responses also allows our brains to think more creatively as it frees more blood flow and resources for the logical thinking regions in our brains – the PFC. So smiling helps us to team up as well as think and be more effective as a team. Smiling also leads to the release of neuropeptides that help neurons communicate more efficiently with each other.

Importantly, smiling even to ourselves, helps – almost as much as if we are responding to a smile from someone else. A 2010 study by Andrew Oswald, a professor of economics at Warwick Business School, noted that employees who smile more often are significantly more productive and creative in the workplace. Combine this with a 2013 study from the University of California (San Francisco), which found that those who are happier have a more comprehensive approach to problems, improving their ability to think of more solutions than their more negatively-minded counterparts. So, smiling can make you and your co-workers smarter: more cohesive, creative and productive! This also aligns with 'enjoyment performance theory', as used by Dr Dan Harrison.

Companies like Google and Ben & Jerry's have known this for years and so have placed an emphasis on happier workplaces (where people are likely to smile more) because they recognise that looking after their staff in this way is more than well-being, engagement and retention of talent – they also get higher performing teams and results (profits) to boot!

As smiling is such an easy thing to do, compared to say, #Tip1 'Cold Showers' and is another 'stackable habit' like #Tip5 'And Breathe' we think this is a winner.

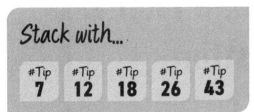

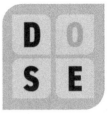

Parting Shot

Want to connect more quickly with people when public speaking? Then just smile! Next time you are stood in front of an audience, even when just waiting to speak, simply smile – as naturally as you can of course (otherwise it can look like you have trapped wind). Then breathe (**#Tip5**). As you smile, others in your audience will start to 'mirror' (see **#Tip41**) your smile and so be smiling back at you. This will boost your confidence no end. If nothing else, many more of those listening to you will be left with the feeling that you connected positively with them – even if they can't remember everything you spoke about.

Aside from smiling inappropriately, like when breaking bad news, it's hard to see the downside or danger in smiling, other than some people smiling back at you, even if just out of curiosity or mild bewilderment. No matter, your smiling will most likely positively boost others' brains as well as your own.

P.S. World Smile Day is 1st October.

Small Moments Matter

The Big Idea

The connection with nature to improve well-being has been known about for millennia. In Japan 'forest bathing' (*shinrin yuko*) is still practised and prescribed by doctors to help calm nerves and improve well-being. So, it is perhaps no surprise that there is plenty of evidence to suggest that improving and maintaining our connection with nature, especially by immersing ourselves in it, can calm us and improve our sense of balance and well-being.

With our ever-evolving technological lives however, we can become increasingly divorced from nature. Research is helping us to understand that this disconnect might be bringing deep and ongoing stress that we may not yet fully recognise. Estimates suggest that by 2050 over 66% of the human population will be living in cities. So an increasing separation from nature may hold some profound adverse health ramifications without some deliberate interventions.

Many of you will already appreciate the benefits of being outside for 10 or 15 minutes a day. Being more deliberate in our lives and enjoying and appreciating moments in the present, to gain 'control' of our thoughts. By combining such moments of deliberate reflection and connection with nature can focus and amplify their effects on us (e.g. #Tip**8**).

So how does the ancient wisdom of being close to nature stack up with what we know about how our brains and bodies work?

Got it... What's the Science?

Our latent 'call to the wild' (biophilia) becomes even more profound when you look more closely at the science. Research has shown that just looking at a natural image or touching natural objects, like those made of wood, actually lowers our blood pressure. And it has also shown that having pictures of nature, as well as real flowers and plants in hospitals actually speeds patient recovery rates, with patients being discharged from hospital sooner.

Architects and interior designers of homes and workspaces understand the power of plants in the room, incorporating them into their designs. Many progressive, creative organisations and companies, such as those involved in new tech, rent plants for spaces and events for this reason.

It seems connecting with nature and natural objects regularly lowers the pressure on our cardiovascular systems – meaning we should live longer as well as think more clearly.

We know that noticing things brings them into our attention and so makes their impact and presence more 'felt' by being in our consciousness (see #Tip**22**). It also allows us to then better control or steer what we want in both our conscious and unconscious mind. So deliberately focusing on nature in particular, is going to bring you physiological rewards that are beneficial for your sense of well-being. It might also spark or rekindle an interest in nature that could be anything from gardening or watching wildlife to painting landscapes – which of course can lead to an increased desire to protect such green spaces for self and others. Together we know these activities activate and incorporate our 'well-being circuits' that use dopamine and serotonin.

And it doesn't stop there! When we go for a walk amongst nature we disturb phytoncides, which are described as antimicrobial allelochemical* volatile organic compounds from plants.

These compounds are known to reduce inflammation and pathogens by raising the number of human natural killer cells. In other words, plants release chemicals that help us fight off infection and illness. It seems that repeated daily exposure has the best positive influence on our body and brain. Just 30 minutes (and as little as 10 to 20 minutes) in a park or green space is reported as being sufficient to start to have an impact, with 120 minutes or more combined a week being to have measurable ongoing health benefits, although there seems little added advantage of over 300 minutes a week. This is particularly exciting as we now know that so many diseases and illnesses, including mental health states such as depression, and neurodegenerative diseases such as Alzheimer's, include inflammation. So time in nature could well be warding off the likelihood of you developing chronic and debilitating conditions and diseases.

Deliberately taking time to be out and about in nature or even appreciate it in a photograph, is incredibly beneficial to your body, brain and therefore also to your mind. It's supported not just by ancient wisdom, but by modern science too, and is particularly stackable as a habit.

*   Allelochemicals are chemicals (secondary metabolites) produced by plants, algae, bacteria, and fungi that influence the growth and development of other species.

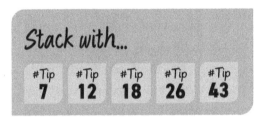
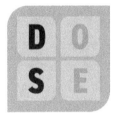

Parting Shot

Human beings are natural creatures so it makes sense that reminding ourselves to re-connect with nature can bring us tangible benefits. What could you do to deliberately engineer regular small moments with nature?

How about a 'walk and talk' in the park as a way to have productive one-to-one meetings or using sprigs of eucalyptus in the bathroom while you shower. Smell is such a primal and evocative sense with direct links to the brain's limbic system, which aromatherapy taps into (#Tip15).

#Tip 12 Playlist for Life

The Big Idea

Music has been a form of human communication as far back as we can trace, and in a complexity that seems unique to our species. As technology has become ever more sophisticated so, it seems, has the diversity of sounds and music that we can produce and reproduce. Today most of us have a staggering accessibility to, and diversity of, music to listen to. Instant downloads and mixing apps mean our musical tastes and how we 'consume' and use music can be ever more personalised.

Most of us will associate a piece of music with significant points in our lives; it might be something you sang at school, your first dance with your partner or a popular song around a particularly tough time. In other words, music can be particularly evocative in inducing or complementing our emotional states.

You will, no doubt, have pieces of music that you use to get yourself into a different zone or place, maybe to increase your focus, calm yourself down, exercise more effectively or motivate yourself for a particular task. If you haven't, this tip is definitely one for you to try. If you have, this #Tip is how you can more deliberately utilise music to get more from life.

Got it... What's the Science?

The process of listening to music is a complex one. Even the simplest melody needs a significant amount of work by our brains to fully process.

Music involves sound being converted into electrical nerve impulses in the inner ears that then travel to our brain initially to the thalamus (the brain information relay centre), basal ganglia (motor control) and auditory cortex. Here these impulses are processed for rhythm, pitch and volume before other facets such as tempo, pace, melody, tonality and harmony are processed – almost extracted – around the brain. Music, it seems, activates and involves just so many brain regions, almost simultaneously and synergistically – including the hippocampus (learning and memory), amygdala (emotional responses), cerebellum (co-ordinated automated movement), PFC (including prediction and anticipation). Many of these specialised brain regions are connected to movement and 'reward centres', which probably explains why we find music both so compelling and enjoyable to move and dance to (see **#Tip16**). And all this before we even consider the processing of language and lyrics!

The combination means that music is able to 'cross-access' and stimulate different brain functions including memory, language, perception and emotion. This cross-processing is why music can be so evocatively associated, almost anchored, to memories of significant events in our life.

Research has shown that the inter-connectivity used by

our brains for musical processing can actually be used as a backdoor way of stimulating higher brain function networks, especially when there has been damage or disorders due to disease such as neurodegenerative conditions like Parkinson's, or structural / processing differences related to neurodiverse conditions like dyslexia.

Our sensitivity to sound (hearing) is a primary sense which develops when we are in our mother's womb. We develop to a backing beat that is our mother's heartbeat. It is not surprising then that our brain is so sensitive to rhythmic beats. We even tend to associate and perceive time in relation to our own heartbeat and pulse. It seems that by manipulating pace and beat we can even use music to manipulate our perception of time. Interestingly, studies suggest that being able to tap to a rhythmic beat correlates with better performance in reading and attention tests.

So what makes music so personal? And why do musical styles seem generational? During the late teenage years our brain goes through a process called 'neural pruning' where the multitude of interconnections between our brains' neurons are significantly reduced to streamline and optimise the processes that have best served us up to that point in our development. So that by the time we are reproductively mature, we are able to do the tasks that we have learnt to do by then faster and more efficiently. This is a likely mechanism or consequence for why music that we were 'into' in our teens, tends to remain our default or go-to preference throughout the rest of our lives. This 'musical imprinting' may also help generations to better relate within distinct generations, helping social cohesion and promoting a sense of belonging and tribe (see #Tip**34**).

The increasing plethora of musical styles and accessibility today means that there is also now ever more opportunity for diversity, nuance and personality within generations. As in fashion, some styles seem to reoccur or at least be recycled with a twist. This is particularly noticeable when it comes to the music we use to get ourselves into 'the zone'. This is in part because the music we listen to is so tied to our memories and feelings as well as the more basic (basal) emotions associated with say aggression and drive.

This means you can create personal playlists that can help stimulate your brain into 'zones' for better focus, performance, communication, even the recall of information, as well as to give you a greater sense of well-being and social connection.

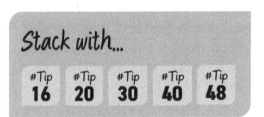

Stack with...

#Tip	#Tip	#Tip	#Tip	#Tip
16	**20**	**30**	**40**	**48**

For our playlist of music with bpm of 120, check out https://the52project.com/tip12-playlist-for-life.

Parting Shot

Our brains' love for music is why, in part, Martin Luther King's 'I have a dream' speech was, and remains, so powerful and evocative. He used rhythm, cadence, tone as well as metaphor, rhetoric and imagery from his Gospel roots to so passionately move his audience and change our world.

#Tip 13 Treat Yourself

The Big Idea

We first considered this tip at Easter, a time of the year where eating chocolate is not only 'allowed' but positively celebrated!

As a result, we thought we would look at the science of why chocolate (in moderation) is good for you and why 'treating' yourself to a reward actually works as a way to feel good and perform better. By now you will perhaps not be surprised that it's all about those positive 'brain chemicals' whose levels are behind how motivated, happy or energised we can feel.

You may have heard phrases before like "a little bit of what you fancy does you good", – well luckily for us, the science backs this up!

Got it... What's the Science?

Consuming chocolate regularly has been found to help the brain function, thanks to cocoa being a rich source of natural neuroprotective compounds. These compounds do what they say on the tin – they protect our brains from the harm it might otherwise come to from the hazards around us in everyday life. You might have heard

these protective compounds described as 'antioxidants'. These useful bioactive compounds, found in raw cocoa beans, are called flavanols (flavan-3-ols) that are also found in teas, apples and several berries. These group of compounds have been reported to also exhibit several health benefits including protecting the heart and vascular system (cardioprotective), and protecting against cancers (anticarcinogenic). In short, eating a bit of chocolate can provide positive protection against some of the nastier things in life!

The benefits don't stop there. Chocolate contains theobromine (which interestingly, like caffeine is also found in tea). Theobromine is a stimulant related to, but milder than, caffeine in its effects, which is also a vasodilator, meaning that it temporarily increases blood flow and reduces blood pressure. A small study of 30 healthy adults published in 2010 attributed theobromine to short term improved mental performance and reduced mental fatigue.

This is another reason that chocolate or a cup of tea gives you the sense of having a bit of a lift. You get a quick rush of blood as a result of having that cuppa – especially so if you combine it with a dark chocolate biscuit! (Generally, the darker the chocolate, the greater the concentration of theobromine.)

There is, however, a word of caution – otherwise all we would do in life is fill it with tea and biscuits! Don't overdo it! According to the National Hazardous Substances Database: "It has been stated that 'in large doses' theobromine may cause nausea and anorexia and that daily intake of 50–100g raw cocoa (about 0.8–1.5g theobromine) by humans has been associated with sweating, trembling and severe headaches."

Let's go with the benefits of moderation because they do appear to stack up pretty well. Like flavanols, theobromine also seems to have antitumoral and anti-inflammatory properties without some of the undesirable side effects that you get from caffeine. For instance, theobromine might actually help improve sleep quality.

Chocolate is also a source of phenylethylamine. This compound stimulates the brain to release dopamine which is associated with feelings of pleasure and motivation. Chocolate also contains numerous other psychoactive chemicals such as small amounts of anandamide, an endocannabinoid neurotransmitter, that activates 'pleasure' (CB1) receptors in the brain (these are, as the name suggest, mostly responsible for the euphoric effects of cannabis). Chocolate also contains chemicals (ethanolamines) that slow the breakdown (hydrolisation) of these anandamides ('bliss chemicals') that are naturally produced and present in your brain. Together these intensify and prolong the chocolate associated feel-good state. It is also likely partly why we can find chocolate addictive.

So there really is evidence to say that chocolate can boost your mood. Researchers have found evidence of mental health benefits from eating chocolate. A study of over 13,000 individuals from the US reported in the journal, *Depression and Anxiety*, in 2019, showed that people who ate any amount of dark chocolate during two 24-hour periods had "70% lower odds of reporting clinically relevant depressive symptoms," than those that ate no chocolate at all. The key here seems to be dark chocolate that contains the higher percentages of cocoa. That said, the top 25% consumers of all chocolate types studied were still least likely to say they experienced depressive symptoms.

We also know that the anticipation of a treat also boosts dopamine release. So the great news here is the anticipation of treating yourself, or getting a reward (#Tip**37**), means you can get well-being benefits just from preparing to have your 'treat break'. All in all, this makes treating yourself an exceptionally adaptable and stackable habit. So, think about where and when you can next treat yourself, maybe in the garden (#Tip**11**), getting some morning sunshine, checking in on your breathing (#Tip**5**) and taking some time to reflect.

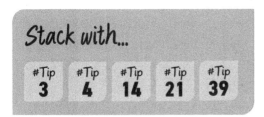

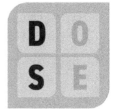

Parting Shot

A little bit of what you fancy is definitely a science backed win! Make your treat as guilt free as you can by getting the balance right. We call that the 'Goldilocks effect' – not too little, not too much – getting it just right for you.

And do remember to take time to anticipate treats too – for an extra boost of dopamine with no additional calories!

#Tip
14 **Plant Power**

The Big Idea

We love that #Tip inspiration can come from the most random convergences. Dulcie, on a night out with an old friend with whom 'beetroot' was an in-joke, mentioned this joke to another at the festivities. The new acquaintance then told them both about how his doctor had recommended beetroot juice instead of taking tablets to reduce his blood pressure.

Having had a fascination with all things beetroot with the same old friend from a young age, Dulcie insisted on trying some right that minute. To her surprise she actually liked it.

Some years later, this night out's beetroot juice frivolity came to mind whilst Dulcie watched a BBC episode of *Trust Me, I'm a Doctor*. The programme was exploring how beetroot juice could be a real natural health 'bullet'. Not only to lower blood pressure but even promising to improve athletic performance. It seems that beetroot juice enables people to train faster, harder and for longer, improving their times over their chosen distances. Not only this but study participants stayed mentally sharper after exercise too!

Got it... What's the Science?

According to scientists from Queen Mary University of London, drinking 250ml of beetroot juice daily was found to lower high blood pressure, and when consumed over a 4-week period, decreased it to levels linked with significantly reduced likelihood of death by heart disease or stroke. Study participants also showed improved health, principally increased flexibility, of the inner lining of their blood vessels.

So how could this be? Beetroot is naturally high in nitrates and these are converted in the body to nitric oxide (NO). These nitrates, now NO, enable blood vessels to further open up, allowing the blood to flow more smoothly and efficiently. Nitrates also seem to have a remarkable effect on stamina when exercising. One study, at the University of Exeter, suggests that in a clinically controlled trial, people were able to train for 16% longer after consuming beetroot juice. This also resulted in about a 2% decrease in the time it took the athlete to complete their usual race. This is the kind of improvements in performance that elite athletes dream of.

The study makes fascinating reading and has really interesting implications. Professor Andy Jones, then an adviser to top UK athlete Paula Radcliffe, said: "We were amazed by the effects of beetroot juice on oxygen uptake because these effects cannot be achieved by any other known means, including training."

While the study was of obvious interest to professional

and amateur athletes, Professor Jones also went on to "explore the relevance of the findings to those people who suffer from poor fitness and may be able to use dietary supplements to help them go about their daily lives."

The BBC's *Trust Me, I'm a Doctor* programme helped us to understand the implications for ordinary people a bit better. What if a glass of beetroot juice helped people who didn't exercise to start doing so because they could experience the benefit of exercise without initially feeling so tired that they gave up? Or what if non-exercisers pleasantly surprised themselves with their exercise experience and ability in the early days? And the mighty beetroot juice benefits don't stop here.

Studies have also suggested that beetroot juice can improve learning and memory as well as mental sharpness after exercise. The research is ongoing, but it seems that it is most likely due to NO opening up the blood vessels to areas of the body and brain that need it most when doing challenging tasks (remember #Tip7 and the benefits of water and hydration for brain function). The involvement of NO as a neurotransmitter is currently less clear BUT seems it might help brain cells by acting as a gain or volume modulator for signalling (transmitting electrical impulses). It turns out that NO is 'made-to-order' rather than stored until it is needed, which makes it tricky to study. The BBC study was small but it did back up this research. They found that the usual 'brain fatigue' or 'brain fade' that you can experience after exercise was removed by drinking the juice around 15–20 minutes before the exercise began.

Other nitrate-rich vegetables, including radishes,

spinach and rocket seem to have an identical effect. The BBC study found that a salad with nitrates in was just as effective as the beetroot juice when it came to improving stamina and maintaining mental sharpness after exercise.

What about downsides? Well, there is a slight shock in store if you momentarily forget that you have drunk the juice later on as it does turn urine pink and can have the same effect on poo too. Also please check with your doctor if you are taking medicine or if you know that you suffer from low blood pressure or have ongoing and / or complex health conditions before consuming pints of the stuff.

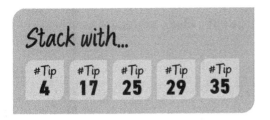

Stack with...

#Tip	#Tip	#Tip	#Tip	#Tip
4	17	25	29	35

Tales from our Testers

Tester, James Bushe, gave us this feedback: *"After hearing the tip I went out to get some. Had a glass 20 minutes before my run, and amazingly, ran my 10km personal best. Even if there might have been some part of a placebo effect in there, it works! It's now part of my run routine, and I feel all the better for it."*

#Tip 15 **Be Smelly**

The Big Idea

Have you have caught a scent out of the blue that gives you a sudden rush of emotion and flash of memory? One that just takes you back? You are not alone! Smell is arguably one of, if not the, most evocative and seductive of senses – widely used to help you relax, to buy, even help you find a mate. For us, this made it a clear candidate for another top stackable #Tip.

The use of scents (aromas) for therapy have been used since ancient times. Despite aromatherapy often being dismissed as a pseudoscience, there seems to be significant evidence that stimulating the sense of smell can be a complementary life approach to even having a better memory.

Got it... What's the Science?

When we smell, we inhale compounds which interact with, and are absorbed through, the olfactory bulbs in our noses which send messages to our olfactory cortex – the part of the brain responsible for our conscious sense of smell. These messages quickly reach other areas of the brain, such as the limbic system, which includes the hippocampus (memory and learning as well as spatial awareness and navigation) and amygdala (associated with memory of fear and danger). In other words: scents, via our olfactory bulbs, provide a fast-track messaging route to our emotional and memory associated structures. So, it is perhaps not surprising that certain scents get linked with specific events, places or feelings. What seems key here is that strong associations with aromas, even from early life, can subconsciously evoke strong emotions and physical reactions such as raised heart rate and breathing.

There could be much more going on than just scent and the sense of smell. Our olfactory bulbs are quite primitive sense organs. Scientists have shown that smelling essential oils containing terpenes can lead to them entering your blood stream via the nasal mucosa – and because the compounds are small and fat-soluble, the 'smells' can easily cross the blood-brain barrier. Terpenes are found in many aromatic plants, including eucalyptus, bay, wormwood and sage.

Lavender oil, whose phytochemical composition (see #Tip11) includes multiple terpenes, is a smell that most people recognise. Many studies suggest that the scent of lavender is calming for many – including other animals. A review of the research suggests that lavender scent may also offer some small to moderate sleep-promoting benefits.

In *Hamlet*, Ophelia says, "There's rosemary, that's for remembrance." That may not be such a wild claim as rosemary plants contain terpenes.

A small study by Northumbria University found that a group of school-aged children who took tests in rooms scented with rosemary received higher scores than children in unscented rooms. A study by the same team used blood samples to detect the amount of terpene molecules that participants had absorbed from smelling rosemary oil. The researchers then did speed and accuracy tests, and mood assessments, to judge the rosemary oil's affects. Despite being a small study, it did show that higher concentrations of terpenes in the blood did positively impact an individual's cognitive performance resulting in improved performance.

Perhaps, like with phytoncides in forest bathing / walking, we have evolved to naturally take the benefits of these compounds through the process of breathing and smelling. This means if we are aiming to simulate or augment these benefits, we need only make small additions like a few drops of essential oil on a tissue, to have the impact that we are after. We all know how overpowering it can be when we walk into the presence of someone who has doused themselves with a potent cologne. So beware: too much of a good thing here is likely to reverse the effect/s you are after!

To sum up, it seems we can be certain that most of us can use scents to modulate our mood and environment to define context. Context helps our brains to best frame then recall appropriate experiences and responses. So by manipulating context with scent we can deliberately make memories more memorable ('sticky'), more accessible and even more visceral. This power can be wielded not only to enrich our own experiences but also to influence outcomes. We are most drawn to scents that we associate with safety, reward and enjoyment. This is why estate agents suggest baking bread or brewing coffee at a viewing if you are trying to sell your house. As well as masking other less favourable scents, it evokes homely safe feelings from the buyers' subconscious.

What positive scent associations could you use to bring you more of what you need?

Which scents could you habit stack with other #Tips?*

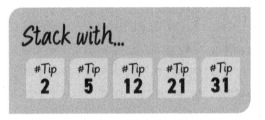

Stack with...

#Tip	#Tip	#Tip	#Tip	#Tip
2	5	12	21	31

Tales from our Testers

"When choosing a scented candle always sniff inside the lid, rather than the candle, as that will give you a better sense of what the smell will be. Some fragrances used in products such as candles and oils are so pure they set off my food allergies – so some scented Christmas candles (and all citrus ones) make me itch like crazy!"

Digital Jen.

*Please be careful. Some scents can lead to adverse and allergic reactions. If you do suffer from allergies or sense adverse effects from trying this #Tip, do stop and seek medical advice.

#Tip 16 **Brew and Dance**

The Big Idea

We all have some slack times in the day when we're waiting for something to happen. Maybe when waiting for the kettle to boil or the laptop to boot up. Well it's time for that sneaky little 'dodgy dance' we do when we think nobody else is looking.

This is a #Tip we got from professional Disney performer and actor, come mindset and confidence coach Amy Leighton, which will help sharpen your brain, mood and performance.

Got it... What's the Science?

When we dance we create an amazing workout for the brain as it connects with the mind and body in a 'neurodynamic' way. It uses several parts of your brain including the motor cortex and the somatosensory cortex that together are involved in purposefully initiating movement and sensing feedback from your limbs; the cerebellum which helps you with rhythmic and patterns of movement, as well as possibly aspects of associated mood, and the basal ganglia which helps stabilise and smooth the movement.

And if we incorporate all the processing that occurs, such

as listening to music as you move (#Tip12), maybe singing a bit (#Tip18) and if you can also visualise yourself moving, being ever more mindful, as you 'dance' through space, you are really giving your brain a full, co-ordinated workout.

The vast majority of us do more sitting and less all-round body movement than we should. Remember, the brain likes and needs to maintain connections and circuits through repeating actions (neuronal 'firing' and 'wiring'). So by getting up and dancing you are keeping that brain and body connection in shape.

You may be thinking "I'm not a dancer …" but that's a bit like saying you don't move. The good news is that movement, including the 'dodgy dance', doesn't require you to be what others would say is a good dancer. You don't even need to remember steps. Rather, just feel and use your body in the moment in some semblance of beat or rhythmic way. We know from #Tip12 that your brain is naturally 'wired' for rhythm, and moving to a beat. According to 'neural resonance theory', this means the brain gets millions of cells across multiple function areas to fire ('move') in sync to that beat. Dancing is the natural outward expression of that beat – even if it is just tapping your foot. Dance, whatever that is for you, is a way that we can all practise being better connected and aligned with our whole bodies for more synchronised action and health.

What's more, when you throw some shapes, especially wide ones, you are encouraging your body to produce more testosterone and reduce the amount of cortisol. Your intentional movement is subconsciously telling your brain, by experiencing (somatosensory) and 'seeing' itself as larger in space (self-perception), that it is confident, even if that wasn't the intention. This means, the more you 'dance' the more your brain is 'told' by your body you are increasingly confident and so you relax. The more you relax the more confident you feel and appear to others and, most importantly, to yourself.

Dancing has also been shown to have other health benefits. Dopamine is important in circuits in the basal ganglia that help smooth out the movements our bodies make. In the neurodegenerative condition Parkinson's disease, dopaminergic neurones are lost. This loss is known to lead to body tremors, stiffness, slow decreased movement and / or loss of balance. Research suggests that dancing can actually help in reducing the symptoms of Parkinson's disease, even reduce the chance of developing it in the first place. We also know raising dopamine levels is also generally pleasurable. As Columbia University neurologist John Krakauer suggests, and science writer Scott Edwards reports "synchronising music and movement – dance, essentially – constitutes a 'pleasure double play.' Music (even just in our mind) stimulates the brain's reward centres, while dance activates its sensory and motor circuits."

Out of the 11 physical activities that were looked at in a 2003 *New England Journal of Medicine* paper, including cycling, swimming and golf, dancing was the only one to have this neuroprotective effect, reducing the likelihood of dementia (debilitating and progressive brain diseases). Regular dancing reduced the likelihood of dementia by 76%, twice as much as reading. This study involved more prolonged periods of dance than the 2–3 minutes private boogie we are advocating but a little and often is still going to have an effect in several different ways.

So movement as dance can be a true therapy in more ways than one!

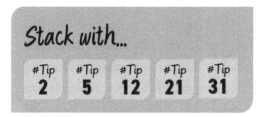

Parting Shot

Dance has so many benefits. Most of us are capable of moving to music and you really don't need to be a Fred Astaire or Darcy Bussell. Nobody else has to see you. As the song title says, we hope and suggest that you can 'dance like nobody's watching' your way to better mental and physical health and even (greater) happiness.

Colour Matters

The Big Idea

How does colour affect you? It is widely accepted that the colours we choose to wear and decorate our homes can affect our mood, behaviours and how we communicate with others – even if colour blind. In fact most use and influence others by using colour every day.

As adults many of us fill our wardrobes with neutral colours such as black, navy and grey. This is likely to be due to an inbuilt desire to fit in (**#Tip34**) especially in formal spaces like at work, where we dress to be taken more seriously as real grown-ups. That is unless of course you are already fully embracing and expressing your inner child and rebel! Of course, you can use both of these approaches (reserved and rebel) with colour – and that's the point with this #Tip – to be more aware of colour and its uses.

Got it... What's the Science?

One study found that people in more colourful offices were more alert, interested, friendly, confident and joyful than those in neutral offices. People in monochrome offices were found to be 12% less productive and 15% more at risk of burnout. And in Tirana, Albania, the mayor, Edi Rama who was a painter and former art teacher, mandated that the buildings in the centre of the decrepit city were painted in bright colours. The result? People stopped littering the streets, streets felt safer, crime began to fall and people started to pay more tax – by a factor of six!

Another study looked at how we subconsciously communicate with colour. People were asked to arrange their entire wardrobe in a circle by colour. Unsurprisingly, everyone had a different coloured circle. However, when those people were asked to choose a garment to express a particular behaviour – to impress someone, or to show you care, people instinctively chose the same kind of colours, despite the range of outfits in their wardrobes. And in the majority of cases, the garment colour was consistent with wider research into patterns and themes associated with mood and behaviour.

The upshot of that experiment is that when choosing your clothing you should actively think about the effect you would like to achieve as you are likely to instinctively select the 'right' or best colour for the job – if you can let yourself go with that instinct (see #Tip**45**). The trick here is to dress for the impact you need or want in the future and not in colours that are likely to reflect your mood now (beforehand) – which for important stuff, like an interview or first date, is likely to be nervous or uncertain. As the songs say, colour wise, you can literally "dress for success."

A study from Kiel University, Germany carried out by Professor Axel Buether, got 500 people to dress in a particular colour to analyse how colour impacted their daily lives. They were asked to document their behaviour over 24 hours and to record how they felt. Firstly, for those of us feeling a bit low in mood, treat grey with caution! In Buether's study people noticed they felt depressed after 24 hours surrounded by grey.

Unbeknown to his testers, Buether employed observers to take pictures of them. It was clear that people actually behaved differently when wearing different colours.

Those wearing BLACK played it cool. Those wearing GREEN were photographed being playful or doing tasks involving regeneration. Those in WHITE were observed being cautious and spending very little time in casual poses. People in ORANGE were seen showing vitality, energy and more than usual levels of spirituality.

Colour is also known to impact our sense of taste – so we can, in part, eat with our eyes. In France, at Bordeaux University, some experienced wine tasters were given the same wine to drink but with some added neutral tasting food dyes. When they added yellow, the tasters were more likely to come up with words associated with yellow-coloured wines "toasty / buttery" and when tinted with red the same wine was described as being reminiscent of "strawberries / leather". Our brains don't seem to be able to cope so well if our taste doesn't match the colour and so in the confusion our brain short fuses – instead bending reality to match the colour. This is again the power of perception. There is a similar but opposite short-cut effect called the Stroop Effect (see opposite).

In summary, colour is definitely something to add to your radar. Wearing it, being surrounded by it can absolutely influence your mood and performance. So be aware, be armed and get some colour in your life!

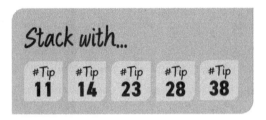

Stack with...

#Tip **11** · #Tip **14** · #Tip **23** · #Tip **28** · #Tip **38**

Tales from our Testers

"My business is called Cobalt Red [where 'cobalt' is printed in red and 'red' is printed as cobalt]. Not only are these my two favourite colours but there is some science behind my choice of words and the colours I have chosen. In psychology, the Stroop Effect is the delay in reaction time between automatic and controlled processing of information, in which the names of words interfere with the ability to name the colour of ink used to print the words. The impact is that the brain takes notice and the phrasing is novel. The more prosaic reason is that people are curious, which opens up questions and starts engagement."

Cobalt Red and Linda Stephens

#Tip
18 Sing it Out

The Big Idea

Whilst your family might not thank you for belting out your favourite tunes, singing along to your favourite tracks is positively good for you.

The quality of the singing doesn't matter. It is the pure act of using your voice that does the magic. Singing helps to reduce stress levels, alleviate anxiety and promote optimal mental fitness. We were helped with this #Tip by professional vocal coach, choir leader and life coach extraordinaire, Cathy Hart.

Got it... What's the Science?

There is A LOT of science behind this tip! There is growing evidence linking singing and improved well-being. Singing is proven to release endorphins (natural pain killers) and oxytocin, which is known to stimulate feelings of trust and bonding and so reduce feelings of anxiety, isolation and depression.

We know that singing, making a sound that is pleasing to us, also leads to the release of dopamine, our brain's reward chemical. And singers have been observed to have lower levels of our main stress hormone, cortisol.

So right from the start we are impacting our brain's well-being with a positive cocktail of hormones and neurotransmitters!

As we know from Cathy's #Tip**5**, breathing is an essential way of helping our body to regulate its parasympathetic / vagal tone (see also #Tip**20** and #Tip**39**) – to help us slow down and be present, as well as to provide that all important oxygen to our brains to improve mental clarity, concentration and alertness. This also helps reduce our stress levels. Breathing and controlling that breathing is a big part of singing.

And there's much more than just a brain chemical release going on. Your emotions can actually change as a result of singing particular songs. Some of that is physical – you may remember the power of beat, rhythm and cadence, including Beats Per Minute or BPM from #Tip**12** – well, singing enhances those benefits. By singing along to faster songs with a quicker BPM you increase your heart rate. Singing along to a song with fewer BPMs slows it down. If you are mindful of your moods, or you understand the mindset that would help you to achieve a task, you can use the power of singing to shift them. A bit like using colour can (#Tip**17**).

If you are feeling low and want to stay low, sing along to the sad love songs. We have all felt the need to wallow in our time and this may be a helpful way of releasing and validating our emotions. If you want to feel better, then stick on a happy song and sing along. If you stack #Tip**10** in and keep smiling throughout, your brain almost has no choice. It cheers itself up by releasing chemicals by the physical act of smiling and singing.

Singing also stimulates our immune system. Studies have shown that those who sang showed higher levels of immunoglobulin A, an antibody that helps you fend off infections. Singing regularly also improves the capacity of our cardiovascular systems which means we are more able to physically deal with stress, making our bodies more physically resilient and helping those with asthma and COPD.

Singing also activates different circuits in the brain and can give our brains a good all over workout. When we communicate by speaking, Wernicke's and Broca's areas in the left-hand side of brain are involved, but when we sing, we also tap into more creative brain functions more associated with the right-hand side of our brains, to help (re)interpret melody and emotion in the music. Amazingly, someone might have a speech impediment but it won't be as apparent and may be even absent when they sing, because it's 'coming from' and involving more of the brain to do it.

We have already touched on how music, especially beat and rhythm, is inherently 'built into' our brains' operating systems (#Tip12) and has benefits of improved cognition, speech and communication skills, particularly during later stages of life. Singing has been found to improve concentration and memory retention, especially in people suffering from cognitive impairment and dementia. In fact, choirs and singing ensembles are becoming increasingly popular in music therapy and mental health treatments including for those suffering with grief and loss.

Those that sing together are also known to share a greater sense of belonging and community, which is itself a protector against social stress and isolation (see **#Tip34**). Group singing can build a sense of community and it has even been shown to synchronise heartbeats, making it comparable to a guided meditation. Meeting like-minded people and immersing yourself into the joy of singing alleviates feelings of loneliness and depression. Working together to create a beautiful harmony will also build trust among you and your peers while increasing your confidence too.

Frankly we wonder if singing is quite simply one of the most helpful, healthiest and stackable of our #Tips? What do you think?

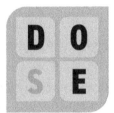

Stack with... #Tip **3** #Tip **12** #Tip **16** #Tip **26** #Tip **30** #Tip **31** #Tip **47**

D O S E

Parting Shot

Many of us think that we can't sing but everyone can sing to their own standard and ability and still get the benefits. And, like any skill, the more you practise, the better you get (see also **#Tip46**). Plus, when you sing in a group, your voice will automatically tend to improve simply by being surrounded by other voices. Try it!

Blink or You'll Miss it

The Big Idea

Our brains are bombarded by information every moment of every day. Some of that information becomes part of us, our memories. There is so much merit in capturing a moment, what was going on for us and how we felt, and our need to remember it.

Much of what we do day to day is lost to our memory. We tend only to remember the extremes of happiness, sadness or pain. Blinking your eyes, taking a moment to take a mental 'snapshot', can really help us to mentally 'flag up' and so more intentionally remember the positive moments in our lives so that, not only we remember them but, we reflect and see more of these kind of events in the future.

Got it... What's the Science?

As part of our daily routine we go to sleep. One of the many active functions of sleep is to filter out irrelevant, or less significant, information from the previous waking hours as instead more salient information is encoded and consolidated as memories or skills. Various stages in sleep then help to wipe the slate clean in readiness for new

information the next day.

So what is the most important information and what makes it so?

This is always what matters most to us as an individual and will consequently be unique to each of us. We call this information 'salient'. Salience comes from our individual ongoing narrative of what matters based on our own evolving beliefs, values and what we hold most dear. These are moulded by circumstance and environment (context). The brain also uses salience as a means of evaluating the importance of the incoming information, whether it is worth paying attention to, whether it 'resonates' with experiences and so whether it 'fits' with our perception of the world. These are our 'frames of reference' or paradigms* which will affect how likely this information is deemed relevant and so stored as 'schemas'. Equally though, events that 'fit our pattern' don't stand out as much, and, rather, can go relatively unnoticed because they are just reinforcing our general beliefs and values.

The real trick to whether something is remembered or not really comes down to how much attention we give it. The more attention, especially if it is associated with high emotions and other sensory information, the more likely it is to be encoded into a long-term memory (i.e. the richer the schema). The subsequent memory usually includes the emotional and physical context of the event, so we can be better prepared to notice similar patterns in the future and so react appropriately (with what worked last time), more quickly.

As we have said before: "where the attention goes, the energy flows". The conscious spotlight of attention is controlled by our PFC. By blinking and taking a mental snapshot, we are using our PFC to deliberately and consciously instruct our brain that the event is significant to us and so to put a metaphoric flag or pin on that firing sequence for the day – to give it more salience than it would have otherwise had. Then when the brain is busy reviewing what to remember in its sleep cycles that night it will be noticed and processed into longer storage in the cortex. The more often these long-term memories are later prompted and recalled the more likely they are to be remembered.

It is important to remember that memory is not like a camera or digital recording. Our memories are incredibly malleable and influenced by the meaning and context that we ascribe to them – AKA biases – often unconsciously. That said, the principle of taking a mental snapshot stands, and if we close our eyes, we are likely to be giving our brain even more space and time to focus on the incoming image, also giving more available bandwidth to other senses and how they link to how we are feeling in the moment – resulting in extra contextual meaning and so salience to the snapshot.

As we have spoken before, our brain has crafty systems and structures to filter and prioritise attention to relevant information in the moment. The RAS is a group of interconnected bundles of neurones (nuclei) in the brainstem that enables you to tune out the babbling noise of crowded room but suddenly pick out, and attend to, your name (or something close to it) being said.

By deliberately saying to our brain that we like and want more of this kind of experience (such 'flagged' or 'pinned' events), we can actually start to 'programme' our brain to unconsciously orient to incoming information that might indicate that a similar experience is, or could be, about to happen in the near future. You may be sceptical of this but try playing this game: every time you see a yellow car, say "yellow car" aloud. Usually, two things will happen: firstly, you will notice a lot more yellow cars than you were aware of beforehand and then you will suddenly start to notice yellow cars even when you are not looking for them. This is our brain deliberately but unconsciously orienting to incoming experiences that we like, have reward or at least consequence, and then consciously noticing specific information. Importantly this affect is even more noticeable if you add a level of fear to what you are looking for, or competition by making it a game.

* See Stephen Covey's, *7 Habits of Highly Effective People*, for more on paradigms.

Stack with...

#Tip	#Tip	#Tip	#Tip	#Tip	#Tip
8	**21**	**27**	**31**	**35**	**48**

Parting Shot

We don't think there are any down sides to this one – other than not doing this lots while you are driving... or too much in front of a first date, or while at a party that is going really well...

#Tip 20 Roll With it

The Big Idea

Digital Jen, one of our most committed testers, asked us to check whether it was true that sitting at her desk and rolling a tennis ball under her foot could reduce stress? You might be amazed to know that the answer is an absolute yes!

And that's not all. A 2–5-minute foot roll on each foot has benefits beyond stress relief. You can get foot rollers on the internet in all sorts of shapes and sizes but rolling a humble tennis ball or even a domestic rolling pin slowly underneath your feet has many benefits including the relief of neck and back pain!

Got it... What's the Science?

The human foot is a complex mechanical structure composed of 33 joints, 26 bones, with 29 intrinsic and associated muscles as well 107 tendons and ligaments. For many of us, without thinking, these all work together in concert to bear weight and transmit force for balance and locomotion. This activity is co-ordinated by nerves running down our legs from the spinal cord, with each foot having around 200,000 nerve endings, meaning our feet can be incredibly connected and sensitive to surfaces, ticklish and even erogenous zones to some people.

Most people wear shoes. In the West the trend has become for these to be with rigid soles that are increasingly cushioned. This might be what the adverts assert we need, but this is not the natural state that our feet evolved into. As a result, some say that this modern trend means we have become 'foot blind' and divorced from the earth (#Tip**39**), so we are less connected to standing as our bodies have intended – dare we say – properly.

This mismatch means we can unconsciously carry ourselves by holding other body regions in tension, like at the top of our shoulders and neck. Working any muscles repeatedly like this, can increase tension to these body areas giving us a sense of stress, which can lead to stress headaches. Our bodies also respond to stress unconsciously by raising activity in our sympathetic nervous system as well as releasing the stress related hormone, cortisol. Higher levels of cortisol increases our blood pressure and heart rate as the body gears up to respond to the stressor. And all this starts from the ground up – literally!

Lack of freedom for our feet can also lead to problems in the connective tissue in our feet, especially the plantar fascia which can become inflamed when stressed or shocked in sudden, forceful movements causing lower foot and heel pain, a condition referred to as 'plantar fasciitis'. Massaging the balls of our feet using rounded objects can really help us give our feet a workout, opening up the fascia as well as helping the whole foot / feet to remember how to be more receptive to surfaces again.

Massaging feet also stimulates the parasympathetic nervous system ('vagal tone') (see #Tip**5** and #Tip**39**), the yin to the yang of our sympathetic system (the parasympathetic is the opposite of the activating / stress activation of the sympathetic nervous system). Massaging our feet lowers our heart rate and blood pressure, slows our breathing (#Tip**5**) and relaxes other muscles and so relaxes us.

It has been known for millennia that our feet have important pressure points which can be mapped for use in acupuncture and reflexology. This is borne out by the parasympathetic affect we have already mentioned, although the precise mechanisms of this are still not fully understood. Releasing tension in the feet can be quite sharp, even painful. This is likely to induce the release of endorphins, our natural pain killers, which can have a wider effect on the body, reducing the general perception of pain.

Quite simply, massaging the foot is likely to stimulate key pathways and circuits that are historically referenced in acupuncture and reflexology charts. The uniqueness of our own individual body, nervous system and brain means that this stimulation can have different impacts on different people. So, when you try this, please be aware that what really works for some doesn't always work as well for others.

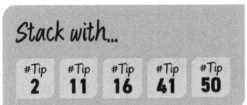

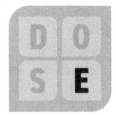

Parting Shot

If you work at a desk get yourself a hard ball (e.g. golf ball) and give this a try. So many of us know that we sit for too long each day and this is a way to make that time more positively productive. Then experiment with a ball of a different size, shape and texture - which works best for you?

PLEASE DO TAKE CARE and start with this tip while sitting down. Hedge Haigh, the professional trainer that brought us this #Tip, encourages us to progress to standing, to give your feet the best all over workout. When you do this balance yourself by placing a hand on a wall and remember to keep your head up and look ahead to a spot on a wall.

We also know that stimulating the foot can stimulate all sorts of key massage pressure points that can have powerful effects on your whole body and how you feel which can include light headedness, sleepiness or a sense of mild euphoria, making it difficult to balance. If this persists or you experience pain or sense of sickness when doing it, we strongly suggest you stop. If this is you, it might be worth checking in with your GP too.

#Tip 21 Hugs Matter

The Big Idea

Of all the things that the pandemic took from our lives, hugging someone special is what many of us missed most. The act of hugging and other types of touch such as handholding or stroking a pet are known to improve our physical and mental fitness.

Physical touch, whether human to human or human to pet, gives us a deeper, more intimate connection that we can't get just from words. When we hold someone's hand, we can communicate feelings of safety and love to one another which helps our self-esteem. Someone touching us is in the moment conveying a sense of belonging, that they approve or love us, just as we are.

Got it... What's the Science?

Our brain's ability to distinguish and interpret touch comes from pressure and temperature across our skin. Each fingertip has more than 3,000 touch receptors. This gives us a sense of physical touch, that is clinically referred to as proprioception. Our bodies have even more pain receptors that communicate information about

painful stimuli to our brains (nociception). On average, every square centimetre of your skin contains about 200 pain receptors (nerve endings) but only 15 receptors for pressure, six for cold and one for warmth. Combined, this gives our bodies a sophisticated network to sense and communicate via touch.

Nociception is the process of nerves communicating information that we experience as pain to the brain – which the brain then interprets as painful. The pain is actually contextual, a form of perception. Part of that context can include how connected we are to others which includes physical touch. When we hug, as well as when we hurt ourselves, endorphins are released. A higher amount of these circulating in our bodies reduces our general experience of pain by acting on both the peripheral nervous system (PNS: before the brain) and central nervous system (CNS: the brain), which together make up our whole nervous system.

When we hug, we are actually more capable of dealing with both physical and emotional pain in the moment. It helps improve our resilience. When your parent gave you a hug when you fell over as a child, or when you rub a painful area, it isn't just about reassurance it's about actually feeling less pain. Carefully rubbing the surrounding area of an injury can help reduce the perception of site-specific acute pain through a process called 'Gate Theory'*, which is utilised in TENS therapy.

When we stroke another, including a pet, our blood levels of cortisol are also reduced which lowers our blood pressure and general tension in our bodies. This not only reduces the risk of heart attack or stroke but also lowers our alert to threat levels. This could be related to a 'safety in numbers' effect: if others are close and connected then an individual does not need to be as alert for danger, which in turn conserves energy and resources for those individuals. Hugging also leads to the brain release of oxytocin which is sometimes called the 'hug', 'love' or 'bonding' hormone because it makes us feel closer to someone.

High levels of cortisol can cause us to have a number of health issues such as lower immunity, problems sleeping and may even increase our weight. Studies have shown that hugging regularly for as little as ten seconds can have a positive impact on our overall health, social security and mood. What's more, longer hugs or petting a pet seem to have very similar and longer impacting effects on our body and brains. This is so well accepted and appreciated that pets, especially dogs, offer a form of therapy used in places like care homes, hospitals and schools.

And if you don't have a person or a pet to hug or stroke you can try a quick brain trick to get the chemical release. If you hug yourself or even a soft cushion, especially whilst looking at the picture of a loved one, you might not get the same levels of hormone release, but you will certainly get some of the good stuff rushing around your body.

---

* Gate Theory – a process by which the electrical transmission of nociception to the brain is reduced at the spinal cord level by the stimulation of associated areas – first proposed by Ronald Melzack and Patrick Wall in 1965 and now accepted in general, if not in detailed, terms.

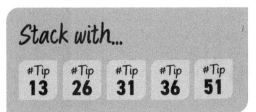

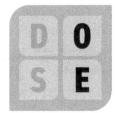

Parting Shot

The power of the hug is such that its absence is felt hugely as an unmet, subconscious longing. Some people feel overwhelmed with tears when hugging someone they know and love after a period of absence. This is normal and releases more of the chemicals in our brains that help with pain, loss and connection with others. Who might benefit by a hug from you today? Remember this is also a mutual appreciation #Tip: you get something out of this too!

This is not a #Tip for all. Some people find physical touch with another person really off-putting. This can be due to their neurodiversity, past experience or just personal preference. So, please do be mindful that hugging may not be for everyone!

Tip
22 Flip it

The Big Idea

As human beings we have brains that are pattern 'machines'. We see, feel, hear, smell and taste literally millions, if not billions, of bits of information every day. To save time and processing power, our brains to fit these new experiences into our existing patterns. We call these processing 'short-cuts', schemas, which form our paradigms (see #Tip**19**) and biases (#Tip**28**).

But what if we can learn to also see the opposite to these short-cuts by flipping our view on something to explore the other side of the coin? We might also begin to think the opposite and so have the best of both...

Our tip is to use a smart phone to take pictures upside down, from down low, sideways, through objects and off reflective surfaces such as puddles - to deliberately challenge the way we 'see' things.

Got it... What's the Science?

The key 'player' or effect in this #Tip that we are exploiting is cognitive dissonance. Put simply 'cognitive' means 'to do with the brain' and 'dissonance' means 'a lack of agreement

or harmony' – or separation.

As human beings we experience cognitive dissonance every day. When we hear, read or see something that doesn't fit with what we already know to be true and believe to be right, we experience this 'brain disharmony'. At this point our brain, often unconsciously, chooses whether this is something to attend to or to ignore. This depends on what else is going on, prior experience and mood, as well as what our intentions are in the moment.

Scientists quite often describe the brain as a 'cognitive miser' wired to conserve energy. It knows there is only so much of it to go around and therefore is quite meagre with it. See #Tip**8**.

This energy-savvy conservancy is particularly relevant if you want your brain to start a new pattern (habit) or challenge an old way of thinking. Such activities require energy, so your brain will literally resist by providing you with a brilliant sounding excuse – like, "I'll think about that tomorrow!" – to see if it can get away with not having to spend energy.

Our brain is so keen on patterns that our cognitive bias will keep looking for 'evidence' that what we see and believe to be true is correct, even contrary to facts that prove the opposite. Our brain wants to do the clever short cut trick of filling in detail that conforms to what it expects to be there to reduce energy and runtime. This is called 'confirmation bias'.

On a daily basis, seeing things as we believe them to be, rather than as they actually are, can impact our ability to solve problems or manage differences of opinion. Our brains, if allowed to run unchecked, can unintentionally undermine our mental health, creativity or empathy with others by going round in negative brain loops, catastrophising predictions or persisting with flogging dead-end ideas.

These negative loops bring with them stress hormones, such as cortisol, and chemicals that in big ongoing doses don't do our bodies and our brains any good. Not only can this lead to us feeling bad, but high and sustained levels of these stress hormones can put pressure on our bodies causing raised blood pressure and inflammation that increases the likelihood of strokes, heart attacks, depression and even poorer sleep (#Tip**24**).

Like any day-to-day subconscious activity, seeing the world the way we do, without consciously and deliberately challenging it gets our brains into a comfortable rut. We know, however, that our brains are incredibly capable of adapting to change through the process of neuroplasticity. Our brains can make new connections in seconds and minutes if they are challenged or need to do so. So deliberately exercising challenging perspectives helps foster greater connections in our brains – making us more aware, associative, and creative.

By consciously shifting the perspective of what we see on our phone pics, and especially on reflecting on what each new angle could be showing us, we begin to appreciate and accommodate other ways of seeing the world and our problems. This tip, we admit, is a slightly tangential way of prodding our brains out of their default 'settings' but learning to see different perspectives from our flipped pictures can transfer to other ways of thinking and 'seeing'. Doing this regularly means we should become more capable and receptive to challenging our set perspectives (paradigms) and so 'see' more of the probable as well as possible before us.

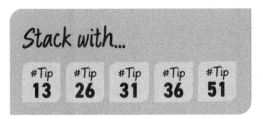

Stack with...

#Tip	#Tip	#Tip	#Tip	#Tip
13	**26**	**31**	**36**	**51**

Parting Shot

There is a metaphysical 'flipping' mind trick that we suggest and encourage, by flipping the situation: instead of what is bad about a situation, what could be good about it? This is the premiss of Michael Heppell's book *Flip it: How to get the best out of everything.* This can become a very positive habit to stack. That said, noticing, and then accepting, that you are going round in a negative spiral can be really hard to do.

Motivating yourself to 'flip out of it' and think differently is even harder – because it requires brain fuel that your brain really doesn't want to expend! If this is you, we'd strongly encourage you getting some help to do this. Challenging your own thinking is often best done with someone else.

This isn't a quick or easy #Tip but the benefits are well worth your time and effort – otherwise we wouldn't suggest you spend your precious time and energy in giving it a go!

#Tip 23 Time to Reframe it

The Big Idea

As Stephen Covey said, "the problem is not the problem; the problem is how we see the problem."* Put another way, perspective alters our perception, and our perception alters our reality. Our perception becomes our reality, whether it is actually real or not. Covey echoed a Talmudic teaching: "we don't see things as they are, we see them as we are".

We all know people who can look at the same situation and see two contrasting things – the classic glass half-empty or half-full. Covey puts these alternatives down to differences in internal perspectives or frames of reference called paradigms. Think of these as different lenses in spectacles – maybe even different lenses in different frames. These paradigms combine to make up our more generalised ways of processing and interpreting the world called 'mindsets' that are often worked out from and in set patterns of thinking (schemas) and actions (habits). These are all incarnated and shaped by our experiences.

Helen Guinness is an international transformational coach and an avid art lover. Helen invites clients to envisage their issue surrounded by different shaped and styled frames which, she says, changes the relationship of the issue for her clients. Helen also says that if we move the frame over the canvas of our mind's eye we can gain greater focus, clarity, and perspective on our life challenges.

* *7 Habits of Highly Effective People*, Stephen Covey

Got it... What's the Science?

This goes to the root of our brain wanting to make a decision about what is there, even if it isn't. Assumptions of what should be there influences what we actually 'see'. This can hinder us 'seeing' something differently, even when we are trying really hard to do so. The more we look at something the more we reinforce the patterns of neural pathways that support the meaning that we have expected and subsequently ascribed to it, upholding the original interpretation (including 'confirmation', 'anchoring' and 'available heuristic' biases). So how do we change the picture and so the meaning?

Visualising a frame in our mind's eye doesn't change the content of the 'picture' but it may shift the meaning we give it. This is especially effective for those who process information visually. We know colour changes both how we feel and interpret the world (#Tip17) so, for instance, a red frame could add a sense of energy or urgency to the picture, whereas a blue frame could add a sense of calm and assurance. Similarly, shapes can contextualise the picture – squares give a definition and security; triangles goal focus and circles a softer feel.

Using a frame can change the emotional charge we

ascribe to a situation. It can also help focus our brains' attention because, as we know, "where attention goes the energy flows," allowing us to be more deliberately aware of what is, or could be, going on in a much smaller field of view.

The nervous system is most interested in changes. If there is a stimulus that remains constant or is repeated, your nervous system tends to switch-off from it because if you haven't reacted to it, it probably isn't that important or you cannot do much about it, so you don't need to pay attention to it. This is called habituation. This can also happen when we try and look at a whole 'picture' repeatedly without different frames to see it through. A 'picture' here for you, of course, could be a story or event in your life.

Framing said 'picture' differently changes our perspective and challenges our internal paradigms and enriches our schemas. It helps re-present the same picture in a new way, so the brain is enticed to see new patterns and meaning. Moving a frame around a 'picture' encourages the brain to 'see' even more, despite it showing less.

When your brain is practised in seeing 'pictures' like this it should make you more creative, adaptive and resilient, more broad-minded and wiser. This is far more expansive than just having more factual knowledge. You can literally 'see' more. It can also challenge and reframe your outlook too. You can consciously and deliberately choose what kind of outlook best serves you, your needs and aspirations – then lean into and live those. Using frames can help you see and steer your life where it needs and wants to go.

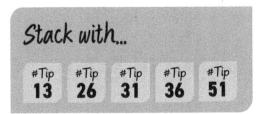

Stack with...

#Tip	#Tip	#Tip	#Tip	#Tip
13	**26**	**31**	**36**	**51**

Parting Shot

Helen Guinness encourages us to try this by actually drawing or writing down your issues or goals, getting out what's jumbled up in your head and putting it down in a way you can better 'see' and manipulate it - be creative here. Once the first draft of the picture is done, then ask yourself what other words, shapes or colours come to mind? Add some of these where you feel they best 'fit'.

If you struggle with making these pictures, how about making collages from pictures cut out of magazines or arranging household items on a surface to represent what you are trying to explore. Take different frames, either made or improvised from other objects, and move them around. Change frames, change the distance between the frame/s and record what you notice. What more are you seeing? What's different? What do you want to keep (or let go of) and what do you want to do with this? You can be the master of your own picture, your own destiny. This is not about flipping or inverting (**#Tip22**) but framing to notice more.

#Tip 24 Sleeping in Sync

The Big Idea

Every day we essentially have two different states: awake and asleep. Our internal clock helps set and regulate our daily rhythms of what and when we do things.

This circadian rhythm is internally set to typically cycle every 24 to 25 hours. Cues in your environment including light, temperature, eating and exercise (called zeitgebers – literally, "time givers"), help your body clock keep in sync with the rest of your immediate physical world – which most of the time runs on a 24-hour looping cycle.

For each of us, these rhythms are nuanced and habitual and are often slightly different, even in direct contrast, to those that we live and work with. So, our tip is to think about your sleep and waking to check in with how well it fits your own natural circadian rhythm.

It is easy to fall into the trap of being always switched on. Without noticing it, we are forcing ourselves to swim against the currents of our bodies' own preferred natural cycles.

This is more than an inconvenience, it can actually be dangerous to others and be really bad for our mental and physical health – all too often leaving us feeling exhausted and resigned to life.

The science suggests that you would be much more likely

to be at your best, and enjoy life more, if you can live a life in sync with your very own body clock (chronotype). Our friend, tester and commercial pilot, James Bushe, was brilliant for this #Tip – given that pilots, especially those that frequently cross time zones, receive training to use zeitgebers to help them more clearly define daytime and night-time and help their bodies to be more alert when they need to be. This includes using bright sunlight (#Tip4) and blackout blinds to nap well… Lower temperatures are a zeitgeber usually associated with imminent night-time (sleep time) (see #Tip2), so pilots are trained to notice and use the temperatures in their rooms during stopovers.

Consider, if you seem to be working with your natural rhythms or against them? Are you picking up your phone when you already feel tired? This might keep you awake when your natural rhythm says that it is the ideal time to go to sleep.

Got it... What's the Science?

Many, if not most, types of cells, including those in insects, plants and fungi, actually have a sense of, or at least are sensitive to, time and cycles that are generally in sync with the seasons including lunar cycles and tides. Our circadian cycles are meant to harmonise with other cycles. In the body these are kept synchronised by the brain acting like a bit like a master timekeeper or conductor by using the Suprachiasmatic Nucleus (SCN) which sits just above where the two optic nerves cross deep behind your nose.

The SCN is incredibly sensitive to light – even when our eyes are closed – which means our brains can set awake-time with daylight hours.

Studies have been done by scientists to see what would happen to their circadian rhythms if they were shut in deep caves, away from sunlight and other zeitgebers. Their results suggest that a body clock can still exist but that their psychological time, based on their unchecked clock, cycled at closer to 28-hour days (including sleep). In another study 15 volunteers spent 40 days in a French cave in an experiment called 'Deep Time'. One subject, in the absence of his usual zeitgebers, experienced days that lasted 40 hours. This shows that our bodies are meant and built to have, and need, cues to synchronise health and function. It also shows how different our body clocks can be from others'.

Not knowing when to wake and to sleep can have serious impacts on our health and emotional well-being. This creates stress in the body, which induces the further release of cortisol. Cortisol and the lack of 'deep' so called 'slow wave' (delta wave) sleep phases, limit our bodies' ability to repair itself and fight infections by compromising the immune system. Over prolonged periods, it can lead to being at greater risk of mental health issues like depression, loss of libido, poorer fertility and increased chance of dementia and cancer. Conversely, timing activities to be in sync with your own circadian rhythm means you are much more likely to experience 'flow' – almost effortless, efficient, harmonious outcomes – when you need them.

Sleep is an incredibly important part of our brains'

activities and has at least four main functions including helping us with our memory and learning, detoxifying our brain, helping us prepare for socially difficult situations and keeping us in sync with others in our immediate tribe (team and family). Our brains are almost as busy when we are asleep as when we are awake.

Better sleep leads to better health, psychological and physical performance, as well as emotional and social well-being. So, this #Tip is to be more mindful of the importance of sleep, so prioritise it more, AND encouraging you to be more aware of and deliberate in using your daily zeitgebers, to allow you to sleep when YOUR body most wants to, rather than when others want you to. In other words, this #Tip is about living more in harmony with your own body clock.

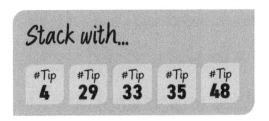

Stack with...

#Tip	#Tip	#Tip	#Tip	#Tip
4	**29**	**33**	**35**	**48**

Parting Shot

It might feel inconvenient to begin with but making some radical changes to work more in sync with your own circadian rhythms could have significant results on your health, happiness and well-being – even your life purpose. If you find yourself regularly struggling with sleep please do seek professional medical help.

#Tip 25 Game On

The Big Idea

Computer games can get a bad press – but it turns out that playing games, in moderation at least, can have lots of different health and general well-being benefits.

We were inspired to explore the power of games after one of our children was handed a special iPad with *Subway Surf* to play whilst waiting for an operation. It was certainly a distraction! As it turns out there is more science behind this than you might think. Computer games can help with pain relief, mindfulness, stress relief and can even grow parts of your brain!

Got it... What's the Science?

Research using Magnetic Resonance Imagers (MRI) has shown that gaming, especially on games that require 3D and 4D visuospatial reasoning, like *Minecraft* or even first-person shooter (FPS) such as *Battlefront* (Star Wars), leads to a growth and efficiency of the hippocampus. Brain fitness and strength, like muscles, seems to require regular exercise and challenge to grow and stay fit for purpose.

What's more, games like *FIFA* have been shown to lead

to lower levels of the stress hormone cortisol and *Quake 3* to higher levels of 'alpha' brain wave patterns oscillating at around 8 – 12Hz (cycles per second), associated with relaxation and meditation. Unsurprisingly perhaps, scientists have recorded different wave patterns, with different types of game associated with different levels of mental activity, including concentration ('gamma' $\geq$35Hz) and the inner focus ('theta' 4 – 8Hz) plus meditative states (alpha) - with differences between the 2 brain hemispheres. In short, brain recordings confirm how computer styled games can help us to relax, disconnect from our physical environment and focus in flow-like states on challenges and games we find enjoyable. A hardened gamer we spoke to, Jonas, recognises the balance between calm and focus especially playing FPS games.

There is growing commercial interest in combining specialised gaming with real-time monitoring (neurofeedback) using portable domestic headsets to especially help athletes and those that struggle to relax and / or focus on their practice. This helps to sustain and reinforce neural pathways that get them into and maintaining more useful brain wave patterns for the desired behaviour. The theory goes that the more they are used by someone, the easier it becomes for that person to invoke and maintain such states at any time – including away from the technology. Literally brain wave training for desired mental states.

Such altered mental states of being naturally affects the focus of our attention. By altering the focus of attention towards games, we can be distracted from attending to painful stimuli (nociception). This means we should perceive less

119

pain as well as likely be less distressed about a forthcoming painful event. In short gaming, say *Subway Surf*, is an ideal kind of positive dissonance pre-op tool or active rest from daily stress.

Computer games have been used for some time to help those suffering from Post-Traumatic Stress (PTS) and Disorder (PTSD). The Games for Change Festival is an annual event that focuses on how such games, as well as more sophisticated virtual reality and augmented reality game like experiences, can be designed and used to give positive outcomes for health, education and relational issues.

There is increasing evidence that FPS games can also provide meaningful and intimate forms of social interaction and identity formation. This can help those with acute anxiety or agoraphobia make meaningful connections online and out of normal social hours. This is why some – especially introverts – found lockdowns helpful (see #Tip34). FPS style games can of course include collaborative problem solving and teamwork which can give gamers some fantastic transferable life and employment skills.

There is of course a dark side to any tool or technology and we should not forget that any tool used excessively or inappropriately can cause harm. We know that the dopamine hits we get from certain competitive binary (win-lose) games can induce addictive and aggressive (testosterone spike) states and conditions that are as real and harmful as addiction to substances – so we suggest enjoying computer games in moderation. Some games that are more ongoing with no defined goal or win, like *Minecraft* or the epoch old-school *Elite*, are far less likely to induce this kind of addictive need and compulsion to win (see #Tip**50**).

So a conservative dose of gaming can help us all to not only distract but to focus on optimal brain states and can even help us all develop our brain strengths and co-ordinations for visuospatial tasks, hand-eye co-ordination, strategy, problem solving, planning, sequencing, prioritisation, time management, socialisation, teamwork, collaboration and much more. No wonder those from elite sports teams, to NASA, to healthcare professionals, to the military and the emergency services are already using computer games in their brain training and therapeutic approaches.

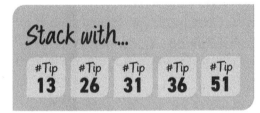

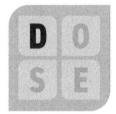

Parting Shot

Our top tip is to find a game that helps with a particular thing that you would like to improve. To de-stress quickly on the go, why not try something like *1010!* or *Tetris*?

For this #Tip we were joined by gaming enthusiast Kimberley Owen who advocates high action, age appropriate, FPS games like *Battlefront* or *Red Dead* to get rid of excess energy. Or if you want to be more sociable, why not try an online escape room or quiz club.

#Tip 26 Ripple Effect

The Big Idea

We all know the warm fuzzy feeling we get from giving, even if it's as small as a cheery wave to someone. Random Acts of Kindness (RAOK or RAK) being good for you is one of those bits of wisdom that just makes sense – it resonates with so much ancient wisdom and family cultures throughout the world.

It is also similarly universally recognised that both the giver and the receiver get a benefit here. This symbiosis requires the giving to be without strings – to be given without the expectation of receiving in kind in return.

Although not everyone will get what we are doing here, together we can be agents of change, to start a cascading ripple effect , to be the change we want and need to see in the world. Where we can pass the ripple on, like rebel ninjas or 'RAKtivists', a term we've borrowed from RAK Foundation website and our tester and regular RAKtivist Jen Rolfe.

Got it... What's the Science?

One of the key chemicals released when we perform an act of kindness is oxytocin. Oxytocin is the 'emotional bonding

hormone' that helps us connect and form attachments with others. This leads to the release of NO, that causes vasodilation (#Tip**14**) which reduces our blood pressure, making us feel calmer as well as giving us a healthier flush to our cheeks. Flushed or rosy cheeks are known to make us look more attractive to others (sometimes signalling attraction or desire). The effect of lower blood pressure, as well as a reduction in cortisol, is also likely to again reduce the strain on your cardiovascular system so it can operate longer and extend your life. So, performing RAK should make you healthier, live longer and more attractive in the process!

A study found that people who are 55 years or older and who volunteer regularly, have their chances of dying early reduced by almost half. Not only that but research suggests that if you give frequently, you are much more likely to be happier and have more stable social relationships creating a kind of positive feedback loop that keeps on giving back to you and those around you. This is the positive ripple effect we are on about here.

Other benefits of giving are an increased sense of well-being and lower likelihood of depression. This is because we know that giving leads to the release of serotonin, lifting our mood. Giving, especially RAK, leads to protective effects against depression. Most people report feeling good, even euphoric, after freely giving their time or money. This might explain why around 20% of money given by 'first world' countries is to good causes from which the givers do not expect a financial return or 'see' the impact directly.

Random acts of kindness are not always an in-the-moment 'fluffy' thing. Those that donate their organs, stem cells or blood to unknown recipients don't just do it for that fuzzy feeling. Research using brain imaging suggests that we use parts of our higher logical thinking brain, the PFC, when planning, performing and generally thinking of doing acts of kindness. This means we can be deliberate and intentional in our kindness and this has some even bigger benefits for us.

We know that we make habits by repeatedly practising circuits in our brain. We know that being deliberate (intentional) and taking notice can make a big difference in our brain and these habits 'sticking' (#Tip8, #Tip11, #Tip19), making them far more likely to happen and become positive habits – so that they happen more automatically. So, the more mindful we can be of our generosity, no matter how small the acts, the more we become tuned into this 'mindset' and way of being.

Acts of kindness are known to release other neurochemicals including endorphins, as well as possible benefits to our immune system. This means that such mindful random acts – or Mindful Acts of Kindness (MAKs) – are the very best way of experiencing and instilling positive change for ourselves and for others, to be the change we need in our world. What MAK could you do for someone today?

For more RAK ideas visit:
https://the52project.com/tip26-ripple-effect-kindness/

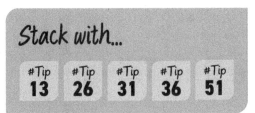

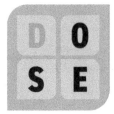

Parting Shot

To be a RAKtivist or MAKtivist consider your acts of kindness as ever-expanding circles or ripples from yourself to those close to you, to strangers, to wider communities and beyond. How about buying a cuppa for the person behind you in a queue, leaving the change in the vending machine, clearing the leaves or snow from someone else's path, leaving a chocolate treat or positive note for someone on their desk. The creativity of thinking about RAKs (so MAKs) and benefits to you and the world are endless. So be the change you want to see.

Celebrating or praising acts of kindness is probably the easiest way to get them repeated AND it's an act of kindness in itself. Don't be embarrassed – make a fuss of the positive!

Random Acts of Kindness Day is 17th February, just a few days after sending love to the one who matters most to you, you can send love to others too. World Kindness Day is also on 13th November and Thank You Day in the UK is on 4th July. How could you tap into these as a newfound MAKivist?

#Tip 27 The One Thing

The Big Idea

We all know that feeling of becoming overwhelmed because our 'to do' list has too much on it and we don't know where to start. And as soon as we start to worry about how much we have to get done, we automatically become less able to tackle the tasks. Focusing on the 'one thing' can be incredibly tricky, so this simple 3-step process will enable you to use that same brain fuel to get the 'to do' list down: Energise – Prioritise – Focus.

We sometimes confuse activity with productivity and expend a lot of energy to not achieve very much at all. Instead, we recommend 'sustainable productivity' – getting into a good headspace so that you can spend a little time thinking about the one thing that will make the biggest difference and then 'focusing like a fanatic' on that single task.

There are many #Tips that we have covered already that help you to energise and focus. In this #Tip, we help you to prioritise, deciding what you spend your time and energy on. Think about the most important things that you want to happen in your future – and then do something about that today.

Get organised! Brainstorm your options BEFORE diving into the first one you can think of. Be active in being proactive rather than being reactive or just busy being busy.

Create a system where you have everything in one place, such as a list or a white board, so that you can look at tasks more objectively and remove the worry that you might forget something. Try the 4 Ds model – Do, Delegate, Diarise, Drop – also called the Eisenhower Matrix. Prioritise the task that will make the most difference – these will be those that are both urgent AND important for YOU to do. Delegate those that are just urgent, diarise those that are just important, can you drop the rest? Even if it is not a task you will particularly enjoy, focus like a fanatic and get it out of the way of you succeeding in what matters most to you.

Finally use Derek Sivers' mantra: if it's not a "Hell yeah!" – then it's a "No."

What is the one thing that is going to make you say "Hell yeah!"?

Got it... What's the Science?

The PFC helps us to attend to tasks. These tasks that compete for attention are promoted by information served up intermittently by our working memory, which includes the hippocampus. These brain structures and circuits have a limited capacity ('bandwidth') as does the amount of psychic or cognitive energy the brain has each day. This sets up a bottleneck where we can waste so much mental energy just keeping the things we could do in mind.

In reality, having too many things on the mind at once limits the capacity to really achieve success. Neuroscientist,

David Rock, says we can only really concentrate using the PFC on one complex issue at a time, as the effort of attention and having to make and strengthen new neural connections uses biochemical and bioelectric energy, and so we tire. Brain science tells us that the idea of multitasking is a misnomer and can be counterproductive, even dangerous to us and those that rely on us. Leaders beware!

You can start to save valuable daily brain energy by writing the 'to do list' down so you can literally get it out of your head and see it more clearly. Using the 4Ds tool allows you to have greater clarity on your most relevant tasks and so it also helps us raise and keep strategic alignment to a goal you may have. This clarity, through envisioning, connecting the dots and planning, can give us a powerful mood boost of serotonin-related brain activation that helps us feel optimistic about the action we are taking, which in turn raises the likelihood of both starting and seeing the worth in doing that activity.

By being more strategic and breaking things down like this, we can get more dopamine hits, a key neurochemical player in our brain's enjoyment and reward mechanisms. This breaking down goals into one meaningful step at a time is a key concept that James Clear advocates in his wonderful book, *Atomic Habits*. Repeated dopamine hits in conjunction with such strategic thinking and action, as well as feeling good in itself, raises the likelihood that we are going to give more resources to this kind of thinking and doing in the future – because we enjoy it and the process of becoming! Focus and reward also mean that we enter more

Task Positive Network (TPN) states that lead to focused action and achievement.

This is where listening out for the "Hell yeah!" (or similar) is the ultimate acid test. The key remains – doing the one thing really does mean less is more.

Stack with...

Energise: #Tips
1, 4, 5, 6, 7, 10, 14, 16, 17, 18, 24, 26, 29, 33, 34, 39, 40, 41, 43, 50

Prioritise: #Tips
3, 8, 9, 22, 23, 31, 35, 37, 44, 47, 48, 49

Focus: #Tips
11, 12, 14, 15, 17, 19, 23, 45, 46, 48, 51, 52

Parting Shot

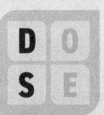

Ask yourself this powerful question, "What is the one thing I could do right now that would make the biggest difference towards 'x'?" Then go focus like a fanatic and get it done!

#Tip 28 Mood Hoovers

The Big Idea

You know that sinking feeling that you get when you get on the weighing scales and they give you a bigger number than you were hoping for? Or that person who just can't help but say how awful the weather is going to be later despite it being beautiful now? We call those 'mood hoovers'! Small things that give you little doses of sadness, regret or guilt. They literally suck the life energy out of you a little at time.

Mood hoovers may seem to be innocuous but left to their own devices they can really bring our efforts and well-being down to levels that make positivity and growth much, much more difficult. This #Tip is about being aware of and steering away from mood hoovers and towards their opposites – mood radiators. Our guest contributor to this #Tip was *Fuelled Fit and Fired Up* author, David Rogers.

Got it... What's the Science?

One of the curious things about the brain is that we are wired to pay more attention and give more credibility to negative things than we are positive ones. It is often called the 'negativity bias'. This bias is so strong that when comparing two people where one is highly critical and the other is hugely positive, our brains will make an assumption that the more negative person is smarter than the positive one, even if that isn't the case! Such a negativity bias is probably to help us err on the side of caution and therefore safety. Be that as it may, this is yet another example of how our brains, no matter how well intentioned, lie to us every moment of every day.

Take weighing yourself daily. When it comes to getting fitter and feeling better, numbers can do more harm than good! The number can become more important than how you feel you are doing and can act as a de-motivator or mood hoover. If you feel you have done lots of exercise and eaten well but the number doesn't initially correlate to the effort, it may make you feel that you want to give up – despite the other evidence that your healthy choices are actually doing you some good!

So when we are trying to lose weight or feel good about ourselves, we need to bear in mind that when we do well, or have a good day, our brains might neatly gloss over that. However, expecially if you have a bad day, don't be surprised if you give yourself a hard time about it – your brain is particularly wired to notice when you fail and / or feel down!

If we can spot ourselves just at the moment where the negative self-talk is about to kick in we can do something about it!

Part of this is to head off wasteful self-critical and self-berating thinking time and energy (see #Tip**27** and #Tip **47**) before it actually happens or is likely to happen. Once you have started to be influenced by the mood hoover, you are already asking your brain to switch away from it – to attend to another more positive possibility. This conscious effort requires the PFC, which as we already know is not capable of doing more than one complex thing at a time anyway.

Switching between one thinking task and another takes brain energy, so even if it is just a momentary, "I look awful in that mirror…," or an "I can't believe I've put on weight," that negative self-talk is something we could do without – both for the chemicals it doesn't release and the brain fuel it wastes!

Unfortunately, an activity like weighing yourself or glancing in the mirror as you leave the house is likely to be automatic, but there are plenty of habits that we know do us good that we can substitute for mood hoovers. So, if it is your habit to get on the scales as your morning shower warms up, try #Tip5 'And Breathe', or #Tip6 and 'Do the Plank' instead – or insert your own #Tip of preference here.

If you reach for your phone to look through social media when you take a break from work and make a cup of tea, why not try #Tip16 'Dance and Brew'? See if that gives you a little boost of energy that you don't get from the phone browse.

If you really can't bear to move that mirror in the hallway, why not remind yourself to give it a really big smile as you look into it and channel #Tip10 'Keep Smiling'.

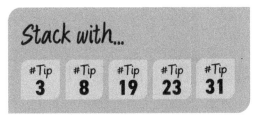

Stack with...

#Tip **3** | #Tip **8** | #Tip **19** | #Tip **23** | #Tip **31**

Parting Shot

Look for the positive. Judge your healthy life-style choices less on whether the scales give you a particular number and more on how you look and feel.

Of course, people can also be mood hoovers. Who are those people that just seem to suck you dry of optimism and your joy de vie?

On reflection, how could you also limit your exposure to such mood hoovers? And what activities could you do instead?

You can create time for these by deliberately and purposefully putting your phone down or spending time around more supportive or positive friends. To quote Dulcie: "it's not bloody rocket science."

#Tip 29 Breakfast Brain

The Big Idea

Intermittent fasting has, it seems, rapidly become a thing. How many social media adverts have you seen for 5:2 (days) or 16:8 (hours)? But what exactly is it? Fasting is going without eating or drinking substances with a calorific content for a significant number of hours. Here we are saying fasting is going without food for 12 or more hours.

The wisdom of intermittent or occasional fasting is actually not a new thing, rather an ancient concept built into many faiths, beliefs and cultural practices – but why? Well, it seems that fasting not only helps you keep the pounds off, it actually helps your brain and body to function better. Keep-fit, health and anti-burnout guru Katie Maycock joined us to expand on why she is a complete convert.

Got it... What's the Science?

When we fast and exercise intensively, and our body has used the available glucose, it switches to another stored energy source: fat. When fat is broken down in the liver to provide energy it releases substances called ketones.

Ketones whizz around our body and can bring significant health and performance benefits. The transition from getting energy from carbohydrates and glucose to fatty acids and ketones is called the 'G-to-K switch' and comes with some nifty adaptations at the cellular and molecular level, including changes in brain cells and their networks that enhance their functioning and improve their resistance to stress, injury and disease. This means that our bodies have adapted to work better with periods of less food (glucose).

Research suggests that you, by incorporating intermittent or occasional fasting, like occasionally missing breakfast, can significantly reduce your chances of a premature death, make you mentally sharper, reduce the mental (cognitive) signs of ageing including neurodegenerative diseases such as Alzheimer's Disease, as well as making your body leaner and more efficient with your body's fuel. It may even make you look younger for longer to boot!

Just to be clear, food is absolutely necessary for all of our health and well-being. But showing a bit of restraint and delaying when we eat, as well as what we eat, can have game changing impacts on our quality of life, as Katie and her clients – and now we – can attest to.

We can start by replacing our first cuppa of the day, that many of us would take with milk and sugar, with a green or fruit tea instead or even just water (#Tip**7**). Maybe extend the fasting period by avoiding the evening grazing habit. Come off auto-pilot (#Tip**8**) and ask yourself if you really want that biscuit or would holding off do you more good than you might actually think? If you need an extra practical step here, practice placing / distracting your thoughts with how this is going to make you look and feel after you have done it – thus combining #Tip**9**, #Tip**28** and #Tip**37**.

This habit also has some other real healthy habit-forming benefits, like making it easier to get out of the 'boom and bust' of the 'highs and lows' of sugary snacks that we can all get tempted to kick start and maintain our day's energy.

Ketones induce the release of stimulating and protective neuropeptides which individually and collectively give cells increased resilience to the damaging effects of metabolic, oxidative and excitotoxic stress. They protect neural cells from 'wear and tear' and ageing. Ketones also seem to improve the ability of neurons to make and sustain synapses by stimulating neurite outgrowth (neurone 'branching'), synaptogenesis (the 'soldering') and synaptic plasticity. These allow brain cells to make the connections necessary for neural networks ('wiring') that makes it possible for the neurons in our head to come together to work as a brain. In other words, ketones mean we can have healthier, longer living, more connected, 'plastic' (adaptive / learning), functional brains.

It also seems that fasting (and sustained exercise) stimulates a process called autophagy which is like an internal hoover system, that safely gets rid of cellular rubbish and debris. This is important because a messy cell is not a healthy cell. Neurodegenerative diseases, like Alzheimer's disease, as well as fallout from traumatic brain injury, are often the result of neuronal cells not being able to process certain debris and proteins.

Fasting, including Intermittent Fasting (IF) or occasional fasting days, also improves our cells' ability to deal with sugar which means it can reduce the likelihood of developing diabetes. Research has shown that combining fasting with a more Mediterranean-like diet (high in fresh vegetables, fish and whole grains, low in red meat and processed grains) can massively reduce your chances of premature death or developing a debilitating brain disease because such foodstuffs better replenish and maintain cell constituents and function as well as giving them stress protection and reducing sources of stressors in the first place.

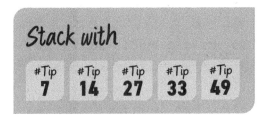

Stack with

#Tip	#Tip	#Tip	#Tip	#Tip
7	14	27	33	49

Parting Shot

Firstly please, please consider if this is a healthy or sensible #Tip for you to try. If you have had issues with food, like eating disorders, in the past, please consult your doctor before trying this #Tip. To be clear we are not talking about overall daily calorie reduction in this #Tip – merely the hours when you eat during a 24-hour period.

It is also important to remember to include regular exercise as well as making more positive diet choices on foodstuffs and drinks to get the best benefits from this #Tip.

#Tip 30 Make Something of it

The Big Idea

Six years ago our friend Jen (AKA Digital Jen) was taking her kids to London and had an accident on a London escalator. Her 40th birthday plans went out of the window as a result of the resulting surgery. Facing a radical change of plan and a serious bit of extremely frustrating downtime, she decided to learn to crochet before her birthday instead!

We were immediately drawn to this #Tip because quite simply Jen thinks that learning crochet saved her brain. She believes that learning this gentle, repetitive skill got her through one of the toughest challenges she has ever experienced. One of Jen's heroes, Olympic Gold medal diver, Tom Daley, uses crochet in between competing as a way of keeping focus and calming his nerves. So we wanted to explore how this seemingly simple activity, could help make someone an elite performer as well as being a lifesaver.

Learning a new skill and repeating it to relax seems to put us in a state of calm alertness and presence (see #Tip25), a mediative state, where parts of your brain take over and the rest of you gets a chance to recover and think more broadly. This can be incredibly useful for people who feel burned out or overwhelmed by lots of 'front of head' pressured cognitive or emotional tasks each day. It seems that doing something in a more automated and relatively simple way gives us pleasure and sense of fulfilment – especially if there is something to show for it at the end.

Got it... What's the Science?

The brain is bioelectric. This means we can measure fields of combined neuronal firing using equipment all over the head called an electroencephalogram (EEG). This technique has been used since the 1970s to measure brain states (global patterns of neuronal activity) and relate them to how the brain functions.

An active, busy, ready for threat, mind tends to show a pattern referred to as 'beta rhythm' with clear cycles of activity running at between around 12–30Hz. As we become sleepy or reflective this pattern slows to an 'alpha' wave pattern cycling at about 8–12Hz. As we enter a meditative-like state we are in an even slower 'theta' pattern at around 4–8 Hz. Theta is typically related to when we do well practised activities like driving for a while or taking a shower. In theta, people tend to report being more reflective, with thoughts bubbling in the mind but with less, or no, judgement, even a sense of mild euphoria and detachment. It can lead to the brain making looser and more creative connections and leaps. Have you ever had a great idea when you are in the shower or driving? It's believed that the balance and interplay between alpha and theta rhythms / wave patterns that are the neurophysiological underpinning of 'mindfulness' and the neural correlates of the 'active rest' or 'flow states' that many athletes and extreme sports people, as well as practised meditators, aim for.

And this is not all. There will be hits from our old friends, serotonin and dopamine, which are associated with looking forward to and achieving pleasurable outcomes whilst doing an involved activity that absorbs us. This is before we consider the benefits that activities and interests like crochet or knitting bring to meeting like-minded people. This social interaction and sense of belonging to a group can also have many protective and healthy benefits for our mental well-being and general health – reducing stress and social isolation (#Tip**34**).

Tom Daley says that he is a natural fidgeter especially when he is waiting for his event. It seems that crocheting for him not only gives his hands and brain something to do, but actually helps calm his mind in readiness for the high performance when he most needs it. All too often those with neurodivergent conditions, like attention deficit and hyperactivity (ADH), are made to sit still and in silence. This is an example of an activity that would actually help those with their attention and performance.

Of course, you don't have to crochet or knit. Similar effects should come from any practical activity that are both repetitive and absorbing such as drawing, painting, pottery, bread-making, icing cakes, sanding furniture, flower arranging, weaving etc. Any activity that requires or involves large parts of the brain repetitively co-ordinating with each other.

The key here is to 'surf' this 'theta' state and avoid entering either 'delta' at 0.1–4Hz (sleep), or moving back into 'alpha' or 'beta' or the much-heightened 'gamma' at 30–100Hz that is linked to intense concentration and problem solving. So, doing a practical activity means we kind of 'mind surf' a meditative state where the activity is our surfboard that keeps us more in 'theta' or between 'theta' and 'alpha' (see **#Tip25**).

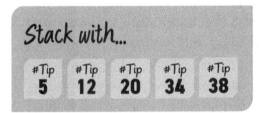

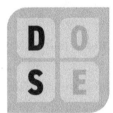

Parting Shot

This is one of those #Tips that is rich for both experimenting and habit stacking with. What activities could help you to mind surf your brain waves?

141

#Tip
31 Let it Go

The Big Idea

Who hasn't got baggage? And we're not talking suitcases! We are talking about the things that we each carry emotionally and psychologically day to day.

It's almost impossible to go through life without stuff happening which has an impact. Some people prefer to bury the baggage, or to lock it away, but this not only requires ongoing emotional energy to keep the 'lid on', it's rarely a healthy long-term solution. Sometimes previous hurts, if worked through, can be reframed and be used as a force for good, as in righting wrongs, but when baggage festers it tends to get heavier. It becomes toxic and destructive to our attempts to gain and keep a positive mindset.

What if we can learn, as a habit, to let some hurts and offences go before they become really toxic? Research suggests that those that can let stuff go, who can forgive, can expect longer and happier lives. Being able to 'let it go' should protect you against you becoming your own worst mood hoover (#Tip28), freeing yourself and others to be more of who you want and need to be.

Got it... What's the Science?

Hurt leads to embedded defensive behaviour on our part, which can 'run' close to the surface of our mind if we are around situations that provoke such a defence. A brain structure known as the amygdala is associated with remembering threatening contexts and is part of the limbic system which is involved in emotions. If we are in an active state of alert and suppression of threat, a big part of our mental bandwidth is taken up with 'running' these defence circuits. This reduces our capacity to attend to other things. It can also mean we hold our bodies on standby, in a stressed state of readiness to defend ourselves.

As the brain only has a certain amount of 'attentional bandwidth', we can find it difficult to fully focus on tasks if we are distracted. This gets even narrower when we feel threatened as blood is diverted from our PFC to our body's muscles so that it can be ready to Fight, Flight, Freeze or Flock. This then can lead to accidents and errors as our diminished attentional capacity means we miss things including good things and positive opportunities.

Pain and hurt can cloud our judgement of what is important. Left unchecked this can be the start of obsessive and ruminating thoughts that lead to acute anxiety and phobias which in turn demand even more of our finite bandwidth to run or try and keep in check. Such thinking raises the salience of the situation or subject of our rumination, which thanks to the RAS, means we end up by seeing more of this threat – and so perceiving it disproportionately as a present and imminent threat, meaning we stay in a state of alertness and anxiety.

Ironically, holding onto things ('baggage') can take up so much bandwidth and runtime, that not only do we lose out to opportunities to be happier, it also means we can be less capable to sense and react to more likely and imminent threats. This is the fascinating perplexity of risk, what is risky to one is not risky to another. Nevertheless, each state is 'real' to the individual. So we need to be more sympathetic in accepting and understanding in challenging each other on them. Bottom line is we need to be mindful what we keep on the bus – baggage has a habit of tripping us all up.

Andy Cope, in his book *The Art of Being Brilliant*, suggests that successful and happy people are those that choose to 'see' the world in such ways because they can let go of stuff. By hanging onto baggage, we hinder our ability to do the same.

One of the keys to this #Tip is being more mindful of whether something is worthwhile even picking up in the first place. And if we do, can we let it go as soon as possible? Positive distraction and more positive replacement 'go-to' behaviours, like smiling in adversity can be very useful and is an approach used in cognitive behavioural therapy (CBT) (see #Tip10 and #Tip28).

Letting go of some hurts as soon as possible helps interfere with the brain encoding such incidents as a real threat. Of course, 'letting it go' can be forgiving someone of something that they did to you. This is a fertile space for getting another brain boost of serotonin and dopamine through RAK (**#Tip26**). Whilst any perpetrator or aggressor only gets more of what they give out on themselves.

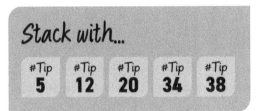

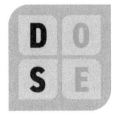

Parting Shot

What might you benefit from letting go? Destructive or unhealthy relationships? Longing for a certain career? The perfect partner? Those old letters or clothes? The micromanagement of your team? That repetitive adjective we use to describe ourselves? By choosing to let these go you can release them, and more importantly, you, yourself, to a new, healthier outlook on life.

Thanks to dopamine hits, the feelings associated with letting go can become quite addictive.

This #Tip definitely comes with a health warning: if it raises some issues for you, do seek help from your doctor. You may also benefit from working with a professional therapist or counsellor to help you. You can find accredited professional practitioners here:
https://www.bacp.co.ukb (UK),
https;//www.aapweb.com (USA),
https://www.pacfa.org.au (Australia),
https://nzac.org.nz (New Zealand).
https://www.therapist-directory.co. and www.c4cs.org (South Africa
https://www.therapyroute.com (International)

#Tip 32 Mind Your Language

The Big Idea

Learning a new language could sound like another one of those activities that takes up too much time and energy when you could be doing something else BUT you could be missing out if you don't.

Learning a new language can improve your overall cognitive function, in particular your problem-solving skills, your verbal reasoning, your attention and short-term memory. Also, it can give you a sense of achievement that we know can give you dopamine hits that are good for your health and sense of well-being. So even if you end up not becoming completely fluent, it's worth giving it a try to boost your general brain power and make you feel good.

Here are our six tips to make learning a new language easier:

1. Do it little and often – learning in short bursts everyday can help you build knowledge and keep the basic phrases fresh.
2. Watch films or TV in foreign languages.
3. Put up sticky notes at home – put short phrases around your house to commit them to memory.
4. Use personalised flash cards and a language diary.
5. Follow recipes in your chosen foreign language.
6. Practise talking about your daily routine in your new language.

Got it... What's the Science?

Language is a skill that the brain takes seriously. In the late 19th century Broca and Wernicke suggested that certain parts of our brain (usually in the mid left side of the cerebral cortex) appear necessary for our ability to create and understand language. For some time neuroscientists thought that these areas were specific and defined. Today these areas are seen as being a bit more enigmatic with about 90% of the population having a left-hemisphere dominance for language. This probably reflects both how plastic and integrated language is to brain function and purpose. One hemisphere can also pick up after damage to the other. This re-emphasises how dynamic or 'plastic' our brain architecture is and can be.

What we do know is that if these regions are 'set aside' for language then one of the best ways of exercising them is to give them challenge. The obvious way in which to do this is to use language as much and as broadly as possible, including reading different styles of writing – from Shakespeare to Tweets and comics. This helps us make broader connections with meaning (Wernicke's area) and the ability to produce language (Broca's area) and connect with other aspects of our cognition, reasoning, memory and emotion. Learning a new language can stretch and so add to our brain's ability to think and communicate that thinking in broader, more expansive ways.

Challenging ourselves to try something that is hard, and

in which we will undoubtedly fail, is part of Carol Dweck's coined 'growth mindset', where challenge and the micro-failures needed to acquire task mastery are embraced, even enjoyed. When we exercise a growth mindset in one part of our life, it can become a habit in how we approach others in our life. So regularly learning and practising using a language can be a like an exercise workout to keep our growth mindset attitude topped up.

Research also suggests that learning a language means that the brain gets better at focusing attention. The more proficient you become at a new language, the more your brain has to work to suppress one language while it uses the other – the one you deem most useful in that moment. As language is so contextual and even meaning specific (some words and phrases just don't translate) this can be a very powerful and energy-intensive process to begin with. The effort of doing this though, means that your brain becomes better at filtering or attending to what it is doing in other things too. What's more, research suggests that learning another language seems to postpone the onset of dementia symptoms by four to five years.

And there are other benefits for the way you think such as appreciating different cultural nuances that give you different perspectives and ways of expressing them. It can also help you to feel and experience the world, relationships and work differently. Dare we say, learning languages helps you to experience and enjoy life more fully? Being bilingual has also shown to help put off the onset of dementia.

Lastly, at least trying to speak the native language

when abroad can earn appreciation and latitude from those whose country we are visiting. We suspect that this works on a mutual respect and a 'you are like us' connection level (**#Tip34**) that can lead to furthering your language skills, as well as undoubtedly helping in making relationships, which bring even more opportunities and rewards. So it seems there is A LOT more to learning a new language than perhaps first meets the eye – with lots of opportunities for dopamine hits from achievements and rewards associated with it.

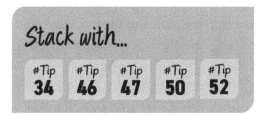

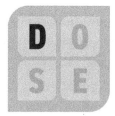

Parting Shot

It's worth bearing in mind that although language can be considered as logical, its use can be creative. Before Vincent van Gogh became an artist he was a language teacher.

Many of us are spoilt for resources to learn new skills, including speaking to native speakers from the comfort our own homes – arguably learning new languages has possibly never been as accessible, useful or rewarding. What language have you always wanted to have a go at? What language apps or courses could you sign up to make it happen?

#Tip
33 Cut it Out

The Big Idea

Do you rely on caffeine to get through the day; to wake up and stay energised? For many of us, starting the day includes making a cuppa or visiting our favourite café or coffee house to get our caffeine pick-me-ups.

Caffeine can improve our memory, decrease our sense of fatigue and improve some aspects of our mental functioning. It can also make us feel good and, increasingly having a cuppa, of tea (*Camellia sinensis*) or coffee (*Coffea arabica*), together has become a go-to way of making and maintaining all sorts of relationships, from romantic to working ones. Culturally, drinking tea has apparently got us through many a crises too. Together, this has undoubtedly contributed to caffeine becoming the most widely used psychoactive drug in the world. Caffeine is after all a psychoactive stimulant that acts on the brain and the Central Nervous System (CNS).

Unfortunately, like any drug, caffeine has its downsides, including: dependence, induced anxiety and nervousness (so called 'jitters' or 'being wired'). Consequently caffeine is a regulated substance in certain professions like commercial pilots and air traffic controllers because amongst these side effects is dehydration (caffeine is a diuretic #Tip7), that can lead to thinking patterns and behaviour that is frenetic and disorganised, which could have catastrophic consequences.

Caffeine also disturbs that most important of healthy activities – sleep – by upsetting our natural circadian rhythms, which in turn can even impact how we relate to others, when and how well we eat, even our immune system (see #Tip24).

Got it... What's the Science?

Caffeine chemically competes with all types of adenosine receptors (it's an adenosine receptor antagonist) – including those in our brain. Adenosine (a byproduct of metabolism of adenosine triphosphate (ATP) to release energy) is present in lots of extracellular spaces and body fluids, and as such is also a signalling molecule that includes helping our body to know when we are / should be feeling tired and so need to sleep to replenish energy (ATP) stores.

By blocking this signal with caffeine we also dupe our brain into thinking that it has more daily energy reserve than it actually has. The build-up of adenosine continues, masked, until our liver breaks down the caffeine to a point that 'reveals' the backlog of adenosine. This is why we can suddenly 'crash' after drinking coffee or tea. To prevent these dips or crashes, however, we all too often resort to more caffeine. This can mean we are left needing much more sleep than we think.

Caffeine not only interferes with our circadian rhythms and the timing of our sleep, it also affects the quality of our deep sleep and sleep health as a whole (#Tip24). Deep sleep is important in our body's ability to heal and regenerate itself. According to sleep scientist Matthew Walker, one dose of caffeine before bed can affectively 'sleep age' your brain by about 15 years. Caffeine is also a vasoconstrictor. It narrows the diameter of blood vessels which raises blood pressure. Reducing caffeine intake has been found to reduce blood pressure, which decreases the risk of heart disease. It also allows the blood vessels to open up back to normal diameters. These sudden changes in blood flow can cause withdrawal headaches. Curbing our caffeine habit and dependence means such headaches should subside.

The habitual consumption of caffeine will temporarily alter your brain's chemical makeup meaning caffeine also impacts other biological actions and functions. Similar to any other drug dependence the effects of withdrawal can be similar too: mental fog, fatigue, throbbing headaches, nausea, and flu-like symptoms. Caffeine withdrawal is even recognised as a mental disorder.

So, taken together, despite caffeine showing signs of being useful in treatment for some neurodegenerative diseases and neurological conditions, habitual daily caffeine can in effect mean we are ageing our body prematurely. If you are keen to reduce or cut out caffeine then we strongly encourage you to do this gradually. Start with cutting out or substituting your last cuppa of the day. Decaffeinated drinks tend to have much, much less – not necessarily absolutely no – caffeine in them so they can be a great way of starting to cut back.

Cutting caffeine out or reducing our daily intake should

benefit our brain and well-being and make us healthier by being more in-sync with our body's natural daily rhythms. It also means that when you really need to use caffeine you can reap the benefits and return to your natural rhythms more easily too (#Tip24).

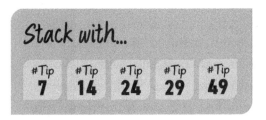

Stack with...

#Tip	#Tip	#Tip	#Tip	#Tip
7	14	24	29	49

Parting Shot

Next time you go to make another coffee or grab another cup of tea, why not choose a decaf option? How about a glass of beetroot juice instead (#Tip14)? Gradually cutting down caffeine will break your cycle of caffeine addiction and dependence. People have different tolerances to caffeine as their body's liver enzymes break it down at different speeds, but the average half-life of caffeine is about five hours. So when cutting back, start with the last cuppa in your daily routine for optimal benefits to your sleep.

Caffeine is a drug and we strongly encourage you to seek the advice of your doctor if you have any side effects from caffeine or reducing your caffeine intake. There is a chance that your caffeine habit has masked other medical conditions. So always take symptoms seriously and act promptly!

#Tip
34 Find Your Flock

The Big Idea

As humans we are social creatures. We generally need interaction with others and especially with those that we most easily identify with – our 'flock'. A flock may be defined as a group of beings that eat, travel and roost together. We are often in several flocks at the same time such as a work flock, a family flock, a hobby or sport flock. Within each of these you can travel through your activity together, roost (socialise/hang out) and eat together. Within your flocks you can share your goals, hopes, dreams, frustrations, achievements and much more.

In the same way that geese and swans work together when they're flying in a V formation, taking turns at the front to share the load, when you've found your flock, you can become happier, healthier, more productive and generally 'better' – there is strength and safety in numbers.

Being part of a flock can also help you find, consolidate and align your own values, even your purpose and personal 'why' – to grow into the person you want to be. As part of a flock, you need to be able to offer understanding, flexibility and trust to those there with you. The value and trust you place in a flock needs to be continually earned or justified – and that's a two-way street.

Got it... What's the Science?

The need to be part of a flock is as old as being part of a tribe, going back to the rise of modern humans about 50,000 years ago. It is quite literally in our DNA. But so is being a bit different. It's this tension between being alike and different that has given our species the ability to connect, to come together, and overcome to survive ,as well as adapt to thrive. This balance of belonging *vs.* diversity gives individuals unique roles and purpose – the real meaning of status – providing mutual or two-way (synergistic) meaning to the individual and to the tribe or flock.

Status is the first part of Dr David Rock's model called SCARF which mirrors the concept of flock. To be our best we need to have leadership that ensures that we can express this Status with a degree of Certainty as to what is expected of us, in our own Autonomous way, whilst being connected or Related in a social construct that ensures Fairness. The more that these conditions are met, the greater the likelihood of individual and flock performance and co-operation. Key here is the resulting reduction of stress both for the individual and the flock. 'Flocking' helps us meet David Rock's SCARF criteria, which in turn raises our ability to think, perform and be a cooperative entity – to be a healthy, thriving flock.

The geographical denuclearisation of families over the last century has increased pressure and anxiety that has contributed to our current pandemic of mental health issues. Studies have also linked this 'dissociation-induced stress' to the dramatic rise in heart disease and cancer in those shocked out of traditionally more tribal families and cultures. Finding your flock will help reverse this modern trend, protecting your health bringing you more health, wealth (in its broadest sense), well-being and happiness.

Finding your flock(s) is an organic process which also means that a flock can evolve, move and flex to meet the 'in-flock' and 'out-of-flock' needs and pressures and give us as individuals both a sense of belonging and well-being, helped along by our internal messengers of serotonin and dopamine. Finding your flock also taps into the need to truly and deeply 'see' and be 'seen' which feeds an innate part of your soul giving you a sense of well-being through the release of oxytocin. Even if the hugs are not literal, these same chemicals and feelings can be induced when we are acknowledged and acknowledge others (see #Tip**21**).

Outwardly, our connections may manifest with specific differences in our appearance and/or behaviour that identifies us as part of a particular flock. This can include what we wear (our flock 'colours'), use of symbols and iconography that includes jewellery and tattoos, to how we hold ourselves (body language), to common language and phraseology (including abbreviations and nick names). These communicate flock affinities to others. Unsurprisingly flocking is a common theme in sporting, religious or practising faith-based groups (#Tip**44**).

As animals we are incredibly tuned into these coded flock signals because they communicate to others a willingness and openness to connect with those that are like us. It can also be a 'short-hand' for us characterising certain belief and values expressed as behaviour that speeds up the process of gaining trust. Trust is, after all, Patrick Lencioni's foundation for any highly effective team (flock).

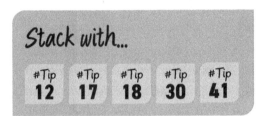

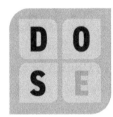

Parting Shot

This #Tip definitely taps into the social science and anthropology of what it is to be human. We suggest that ignoring it is denying you being the person who can get the most out of life and more importantly, the life you want and need. Flocks can bring out the best in others, ourselves and each other. They can of course do the opposite too.

Which flocks do you belong to? What affinities do you identity with from a band, music, style, sport, hobby or faith? How do you signal your flock(s) to others? What contributions do, or could, these make to being you?

"True belonging is the spiritual practice of believing in and belonging to yourself so deeply that you can share your most authentic self with the world and find sacredness in both being a part of something and standing alone in the wilderness. True belonging doesn't require you to change who you are; it requires you to be who you are." Brené Brown in *Braving the Wilderness: The Quest for True Belonging and the Courage to Stand Alone.*

#Tip 35 Bookend Your Day

The Big Idea

How much of your day do you take for granted? How can you make sure that you start and end a day with a sense of your own purpose, creating and maintaining the energy to make life work for you? This #Tip is about being more deliberate in how you structure your day, especially at the start and end, the morning and evening routines that become the 'bookends' of a more successful, fulfilled life.

The great news is that there is no right or wrong way to do this, instead it will depend on your own preferences and type of body clock (chronotype) that you have (#Tip24). Whether you're a morning lark, a night owl, or a shift worker, there are some common things that we can all do to bookend our days. Exactly how, what and when is really up to your creativity and what works for you. They can be very simple activities or routines too. Ultimately your daily bookends become what you need them to be.

Got it... What's the Science?

The key to the science is in how we change, notice and better intentionally value the rhythm of our day, to better appreciate what we have done and anticipate what we can or will do. This positive framing actually helps determine what is likely in terms of performance and fulfilment throughout the intervening time. This is another way to positively tap into how we see the world as we are, rather than as it is (#Tip23).

There is a military term: "fail to plan, then plan to fail." By creating a daily plan which gives us a structure of a good start and end of day, whatever that is to you (e.g. #Tip2, #Tip4, #Tip6, #Tip12 etc.), means we can feel calmer through the intervening turbulence of the day. Getting a sense of well-being and satisfaction at the start of the day can provide serotonin and dopamine boosts that not only makes us feel better but makes our outlook on the day more positive. Inwardly and outwardly this gives us resilience.

Kick-start your day positively, no matter how small a thing, so that no matter what else happens, you will have the security of achieving at least one positive thing. No-one can take this away from you once you have done it. Having something/s to look forward to at the close of your day also adds a sense of security and certainty in where you will 'land'. Remember, that being more relaxed means having more PFC cognitive bandwidth during the day too.

Having a clear start and end to the day also helps with setting our bodies' circadian rhythms (#Tip24). It can be all too easy these days to get into the habit of just expecting to stop and switch off at the end of the day especially with virtual access to work 24/7. This is not how our bodies have evolved. We are meant to have time that allows us to decompress before entering into the sleep part of our days. Providing clear, predictable zeitgebers sets us up to be at our best.

Slowing down and decompressing as a habit at the end of the day can include reflecting on the day and what you have achieved. A study looking at productivity found that just 10–15 minutes spent on reviewing what was achieved in a working day had over 20% increase in productivity in subsequent days compared to colleagues who did not have this time. Putting down your thoughts onto paper, to capture the highlights as well as the challenges, help keep these in perspective and give 'substance' or 'labels' to the feelings (#Tip3). This in turn means that desired connections are reinforced so that learning can better occur and positive habits better form. Tailing a day in this way can help round off and close the door and let go of less desirable occurrences, thoughts or feelings, stopping them bleeding into the next day/s (retroactive interference) (see also #Tip31). Simply talking about the day with a close friend or partner should give some of these benefits too.

Another amazing thing happens when we do such starting and summing up exercise towards the end of our day, we place mental markers in our mind's narrative of the day which our brains will pick up as we sleep (see #Tip19). The process of sleep includes consolidating memories that are significant. By recalling and processing them during the day, we help our brain to remember them in context (see #Tip23). This process is associated with brain firing called 'sleep spindles' present in the earlier stages of non-REM (non-dreaming) sleep cycles.

If nothing else, bookending simply helps us close the day and start tomorrow as a new day.

Stack with...

#Tip	#Tip
3	9

#Tip	#Tip	#Tip	#Tip	#Tip
10	19	45	48	50

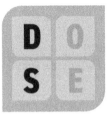

Parting Shot

'Bookending' is one of the best ways to structure your day, partly because the beginning and end of the day are times where you generally have most control over and flexibility – so they can be more about, and just for, you. Which #Tips could you use to set you up for the start of the day and mark the end?

Once you have a morning and evening routine, consistency in activity, time of day and its execution is key. This makes it a habit and a habit stack that is likely to stand the test of time and give you more better days.

#Tip 36 Managing Monsters

The Big Idea

We all have 'monsters' in our lives. We are not talking literally, of course, nor are we talking about the cute and cuddly ones, e.g., Disney's *Monsters Inc.* We mean the darkest part of our temperament which we would rather ignore and pretend we don't have hidden. But these monsters like to strut their stuff, usually triggered by an event or circumstances and they can be difficult to tame. Left to their own devices they can create some rather unpleasant outcomes. This is why we thought that monsters and how to better manage them, especially your 'advice monster' – one of the most stealthy and destructive monsters – is such an important #Tip.

Many of us when asked our opinion by family, friends or colleagues take this as the cue to give them our advice, direct and undiluted from the mouth of our own wisdom and experience. This is giving in to our 'advice monster' and falling into the 'advice trap' that Michael Bungay Stanier so brilliantly talks about in his books.

Our advice monster feeds off assumptions and half-put-together facts that don't really help the people we are talking with. It tends to actually deny others the opportunity to grow themselves, to find better solutions to their challenges, in ways that are far more likely to have success and meaning for them. What's more, most of the advice we ever give is actually ignored and so a complete waste of our breath and time.

A better way is to learn to tame your advice monster by asking more questions. Questions that are full of curiosity and devoid of judgement. Taming your advice monster like this can make you a better parent, teacher, teammate, partner, friend and leader.

Got it... What's the Science?

These monsters are created because our brains lie to us, constantly. Our brains have evolved to deal with the deluge of data we are exposed to everyday by filtering for information that is likely, from our experience, to get us the best fit result most quickly. These filters are the sum of biases that are born out of our life experience and operate at a subconscious level. They are our brain's short-cuts (schemas) which aim to help us make quicker decisions more effectively but they are innately based on partial data that has been interpreted by our own filters (paradigms), to give us a good enough fit for us, in our own contexts. And, as far as our brains go, our perception is not only our reality, but what we think other people's realities are too. This is a huge assumption! The biggest problem here is that our brains are trying to short-cut the very process that really needs to happen for someone else for themselves – using their own thinking.

The darker side of the advice monster is control. We find it much less frightening if someone approaches an issue in the same way we do. It validates our own actions whilst simultaneously robbing someone else of their capacity to come up with their own, probably better, at least for them, way of doing something. This fear response leads to closed off thinking because there is less blood flow to the PFC. Fear also tends to be a state we try and avoid so, protecting ourselves from the fear of opening ourselves up to criticism means we prefer to give ('transmit') advice.

Unfortunately, command and control are still seen as characteristics of an ultimate leader. Thought leaders in business, such as David Rock and Michael Bungay Stanier, have realised how damaging this process is, where the advice monster actually robs organisations, teams and families of the creativity, diversity, connection and capacity that could be released if only more 'advice monsters' could be tamed. David Rock calls this 'quiet leadership', Michael Bungay Stanier calls this 'the coaching habit'. By simply asking an authentic open question we open up creativity and possibility as well as deeper, more trusting, connections with others. We also reduce the stress and limited thoughts that others can have when our advice triggers their threat responses (Fight, Flight, Freeze or Flock). Think back to the last time someone gave you advice: honestly what was your first emotional response?

Mark Fritz also speaks to how an advice-driven leader is one that not only better be right all of the time but is also more often than not the rate-limiting factor in the organisation. In other words, the businesses of autocratic leaders are limited in how productive, efficient, flexible and resilient they can be – because they can only go as fast or be as good as their leader can. Not only do these leaders tend not to be liked and are less respected, they are also the ones that burn out more quickly and have a higher turnover of staff. All this because they keep feeding their advice monster rather than challenging, managing and taming it by asking some simple curiosity led questions.

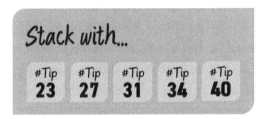

Stack with...

#Tip	#Tip	#Tip	#Tip	#Tip
23	27	31	34	40

Parting Shot

Some say that the mightiest weapon is the pen. We think it's questions. Be aware and prepared for when your advice monster tries to dress up advice as a question.

Such 'solutionising' questions are wolves in sheep's clothing i.e. they are still from your advice monster. So, instead, make sure your questions are intended to help you understand others. Stay curious for longer. To paraphrase Stephen Covey in his book *7 Habits of Highly Effective People*, unfortunately too many of us speak, including asking questions, in order to speak more, rather than genuinely understand and open up understanding and opportunities.

#Tip 37 Wait for it

The Big Idea

We live in an ever-immediate society where everything is ever more accessible at any time of the day or night. Gone are the days when we would go to a library to look up information or regularly write and wait for a letter from a correspondent. This caused us to wonder if we are losing something, after all we didn't evolve to have everything 'on tap', all of the time.

Some of our testers have told us that a top #Tip for them is to delay the point of having something that they like. This gives them something to look forward to and, when they do indulge in their treat or reward, it's all the better for it.

One such treat that we really rate is planting bulbs as we approach the Autumn, taking time to plan and invest in the future. This made us think about our health, in particular how waiting for treats or rewards in the future, can help with our well-being in the here and now.

Got it... What's the Science?

Several studies have recorded the reduction in cortisol following a period of time in nature, and in particular

gardening (#Tip11). So, the nature part of this #Tip is covered but what about the waiting part?

There is a complex circuit in the brain involving the 'dopamine axis' running from the Ventral Tegmental Area (VTA) (a region associated with curiosity), the Nucleus Accumbens (NAC) (a key structure in mediating emotional and motivation processing, modulating reward and pleasure processing) and the subcortical and cortical brain regions which projects to motor-related structures (guiding goal-directed behaviours). In short: we have brain architecture intended for just this kind of deferring, waiting, even planning for, reward – and biology doesn't tend to have such things without reason or function. This circuitry needs to be mature for us to behave as grown-ups, so, not having a tantrum when we're not allowed to leave work early or not binge eating chocolate just because it's there.

We can all practise delaying behaviours, which in turn strengthens brain wiring that will give broader resilience if things don't work as quickly as we'd hoped. Like any exercise, such practice will lead to improvements and efficiencies in achieving the desired results. In this case calmness, patience and self-control. These in turn mean you can make more considered responses to situations, allowing you to be more strategic and efficient in your responses. Again behaviour we attribute to resilience or being resilient.

Your adult brain's circuitry knows it can put something off for greater rewards in the future and this circuitry, if exercised and strengthened, could also help you 'urge surf' the impulse to react to frightening or uncomfortable stimuli such as phobias. By putting off the 'knee jerk' impulse reaction, you are preparing yourself to be more capable and less affected by the stimulus in the future. This is part of many a CBT approach. By challenging yourself to resist impulses, you can take more deliberate and measured control of your behaviour which can be incredibly freeing and empowering.

So planting bulbs helps us to exercise these key circuits and wiring – making them stronger. There is also some more holistic benefits for us here too. Planting bulbs (or any seeds) is a practice of faith and hope for something yet to come – something positive, delightful, rewarding, even fruitful. Something to look forward to. This is an important counter to depressive thoughts where we can feel the future is not going to be better than the now. Remember, we are generally predisposed to seeing the worst and what could go wrong (#Tip28 'Mood Hoovers').

Looking forward to a reward can also help the sensation of actually enjoying the treat when you receive it, because you have been able to visualise what enjoyable things might happen. The power of your mind means you can actually enjoy what you think you might get as well as the thing itself (#Tip9 'Time Travel'). It also means that your brain will pre-empt things to look for that could be related and so raise the likelihood we will get it too. This means our focus and enjoyment can be broadened to related stimuli or objects (remember the RAS?) which can raise the general sense of well-being and mood that we know is associated with increased serotonin.

The rewards for this #Tip probably owes something to

this being an intentional practice that brings about the kind of positive changes we enjoy – an autonomy. This is another powerful antidote to depressive thoughts of inadequacy, helplessness and uselessness. Instead, we can feel we can actually make a positive difference and look forward to that future. And all from the lowly act of planting bulbs (or seeds)!

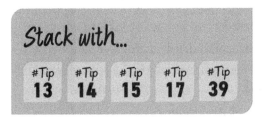

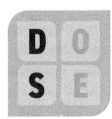

Parting Shot

Unlike some of our tips this does require a small investment for the bulbs but it doesn't have to be money necessarily. There are plenty of seed and bulb swap groups that tend to pop up in Autumn. Check social media or maybe consider starting one? It can be simple as a box that you leave for others to collect and drop off seeds and bulbs.

And you don't need a big garden – a window box or even indoor pots will do.

#Tip 38 Be Abstract

The Big Idea

Throughout The 52 Project we have seen many #Tips where something simple and relatively inexpensive has mental fitness and brain boosting benefits that go way beyond what we might imagine from them. This is definitely the case with doing some abstract painting!

As a child, how often did you paint or draw? How often were you encouraged by the adults around you to 'play' with paints, from getting the paraphernalia organised to proudly displaying your art efforts on the fridge?

Now, as an adult, when did you last get some paints out and just play with them for the sheer fun of it? You won't be on your own if the answer is 'hardly ever' or 'actually never'.

Some of us may have tried some adult colouring in recent years as a mindfulness activity, but very few of us will have done something that we probably did daily as a child – and in missing that, we have been missing an opportunity to let our brains go and grow. Painting in the carefree way that we did as children, provides both an opportunity for relaxation and for the strengthening and formation of new, more creative and inspired brain connections.

What excuse might you make not to have a play with some paints? What 'lies' would you tell yourself about the effort, time or reasonableness of allowing yourself to relive a simple pleasure you enjoyed as a child?

As we know, our brains are primed to find reasonable sounding but entirely untrue reasons to avoid things that feel like an unnecessary expenditure of thinking and effort such as:

"I don't have any of the kit..."; "I'm too busy..."; "I can't be doing with the mess..."; "I'm rubbish at painting..."

But cheap art supplies are available in most shopping centres, and we would happily create a mess when cooking a meal or doing some other 'grown-up' activity. The beautiful thing about creating 'art' is that it doesn't have to appeal to anyone but yourself.

Knowing the hidden brain benefits of creating art makes the end result less relevant. By all means, paint over your first attempt or build on it but perhaps don't write it off as child's play – certainly until you have read the science that tells us why it is positively good for you to play with paint!

Got it... What's the Science?

There is something rather fabulous about what painting, doodling or other forms of creative expression do brain-wise. It puts us into a 'theta wave' brain state with a little dose of serotonin, but it is also really good for creative thinking and problem-solving (#Tip**30**). Sometimes when we don't 'think' we can actually free our brains up to 'think' more expansively, to dream, to make more random creative connections. It's a strange phenomenon, but when you

are not thinking about the thing you need to think about directly, and put yourself into a theta state instead, you are creating ways for your brain to see things differently. Put simply, doing some painting strengthens your ability to think about much more than the creation on the canvas.

Have you ever experienced that phenomenon when you have a problem? As soon as you stop thinking about it and do something else, like have a shower, eating pie, the answer just seems to pop into your mind from nowhere? Brain science at its best! If we know what is actually going on in our brains, we can use this seemingly random occurrence, which is not random at all, to our advantage. This is simple to try. If you want to solve a problem, literally get some crayons, pens or paint and have a play. This should put you into a relaxed theta state and an answer may come more easily to you.

The same happens when we doodle. So, before you scold your child for drawing pictures alongside their homework or indeed a colleague if they are drawing eyes or trees alongside their meeting notes, think again – they are likely to be subconsciously, possibly inadvertently, releasing their thinking and association capacity, that can lead to richer learning and more creative applications.

And beware of the power of the messages and stories we tell ourselves (#Tip**47**). Before you tell yourself "I am not an artist" ask, what actually is the definition of an 'artist'? These messages are not real or absolute and they can prevent us from doing the very things that might actually give us pleasure or bring us brain and wider health and well-being benefits.

Stack with...
#Tip **11** #Tip **12**
#Tip **15** #Tip **17** #Tip **18** #Tip **48** #Tip **50**

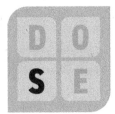

Parting Shot

Borrow your child's kit and have a play when they are not looking or, even better, join in when they are!

When you are next out shopping, treat yourself to some art supplies. You don't need an easel – literally a medium sized pad or canvas and a starter pack of paints and a brush will more than do the job.

Paint something you see in nature (**#Tip11**) and in doing so, you are likely also to be giving yourself a shot of the benefits of playing with colour (**#Tip17**).

The power of play is something we explore further in **#Tip50**.

#Tip 39 Keep Your Feet on the Ground

The Big Idea

Walking barefoot on the grass at a picnic or getting sand between your toes on the beach feels nice but it seems that it is also scientifically evidenced to improve our health and well-being.

But there is more to walking barefoot outside than just experiencing nature – and it is all to do with the subtle interactions of our own bioelectric fields with that of the earth itself. As well as other contributors like reflexology, as we looked at in **#Tip20** 'Roll With it'.

When bare footed we are directly connecting with our environment. Connecting to objects in balance and/or in motion, such as surfing and slacklining is generally enjoyable, despite being challenging, and this stimulates and heightens our bodies' sense of balance.

So, try just taking your shoes off and walk the last tiny bit of your journey home – even walking on concrete counts!

Got it... What's the Science?

Do a quick internet search on 'grounding' and you will find many advocates who suggest that as well as connecting

you with nature and your surroundings and making you more mindful of your walking, it also reduces inflammation, pain, improves sleep, helps autoimmune conditions and improves wound healing. There is also a suggestion that our metabolic activity is changed to such an extent after 40 minutes of having our feet on the ground with our shoes off, that there may be anti-ageing benefits or that it may help prevent or treat some chronic illnesses. It sounds too good or too 'hippy' to be real, you say?

Many of the studies done on grounding are admittedly small and usually done indoors – which sounds a bit weird given that the benefits come from a connection with the Earth itself! However, researchers report observing and reading differences between volunteers that were actually earthed via a wire *vs.* those that were just wired up to an insulated (non-earthed) terminal.

The proposed science behind what might be going on is that everything in the world is made of atoms. Atoms are made up of positively charged protons and negatively charged electrons that come as a pair. So, atoms are generally neutral in charge terms – the positive protons and negative electrons cancel each other out.

Sometimes atoms can lose or gain an electron creating 'free radicals'. Free radicals adversely alter the lipids, proteins and DNA that make up our cells and organs and so can trigger a number of human diseases and conditions. We naturally make free radicals in our bodies through daily metabolism, usually oxygen or nitrogen reactive compounds, but a number of factors means that we can make and / or retain more, such as when we are stressed or exposed to chemicals or certain disease states. You may be aware that antioxidants in fruit and vegetables can neutralise these 'baddies' (#Tip14). A balance between antioxidants and free radicals is necessary for the proper physiological function of our bodies. To remain suitably 'neutralised'.

The Earth's surface is negatively charged and, therefore, is a constant source of electrons. At a simple level it would appear that the unpaired electrons that are on the Earth's surface could partner with our positive ion free radicals and make them less dangerous for us. We change our overall electrical charge by taking on electrons from the Earth which neutralises excessive positively charged components of our body's cells and intercellular biology. As we can change charge quickly when earthing, the assumption is that this is happening throughout the body, rather than just a change in conductance at the skin level. That said, the lack of obvious routes or mechanisms for this whole-body electron sharing is one of the key objections of sceptics. It is also important to note here that electrons do not flow through our nervous system like they do in household wiring.

Grounding research has linked to regulating our automatic nervous system and keeping our circadian rhythms in sync (see #Tip24). Grounding and the mechanical stimulation of walking on the ground, is also known to stimulate the vagus nerve (the 10th cranial nerve and largest in the autonomic nervous system) and improve so called 'vagal tone', the neurological 'calming' tone, which helps you to relax faster during and after stressful events (see #Tip5 and #Tip20). In contrast a weak vagal tone is associated with chronic inflammation, and such inflammation is associated with health conditions from heart disease and cancers to depression and anxiety.

In one study just a single grounding session lasting two hours reduced inflammation and improved blood flow. In another study, grounding was shown to improve the resilience to stress for premature babies who were incubated – decreasing their risk of dying.

So, although some of the mechanisms of action are still in debate, the outcomes of just taking your shoes and socks off can be pretty impressive! What are you waiting for?

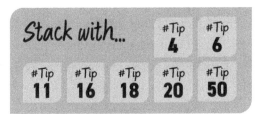

Stack with...

#Tip **4** #Tip **6**

#Tip **11** #Tip **16** #Tip **18** #Tip **20** #Tip **50**

Parting Shot

Try integrating this habit into the everyday, such as putting the washing out to dry barefoot or doing a bit of light weeding with your shoes off to see if it helps you feel less stressed or improves any aches and pains.

Do watch where you are going though and do take care not to tread on anything sharp or in anything unpleasant.

Gaze

The Big Idea

As the nights draw in, our thoughts turn to our fascination with star gazing.

Evidence and artefacts show that appreciating and finding meaning in the heavens is as old as our history, from the Stone Age to early Chinese dynasties, Greek thinkers, Egyptians, Mayans, the Renaissance, right up to modern day science with space-based telescopes. Throughout history the stars have had practical uses such as navigation and calendar creation. And as an activity, especially if combined with some of our other #Tips, star gazing has the potential to be very beneficial to our well-being too.

Got it... What's the Science?

The very act of looking up is associated with feelings of well-being and optimism. Doing this, even when we are having a bad day, can help dupe our body into feeling more positive. The longer we look into the night sky, the more our eyes adapt to the lower light, allowing us to see more – and the more that we wait, the more we see (related to *#Tip22*, *#Tip23* and *#Tip37*).

The speed of light is just under 300,000 kilometres per second. This means that we are always looking at stars and other celestial bodies as they were in the past. The light from Jupiter takes between 35 and 52 minutes to reach us depending on its relative position to Earth at the time. Light from other early visible stars such as Vega takes 28 years! Light from the Andromeda galaxy, just visible with the naked eye on a clear night with low light pollution, has taken 2.5 million years to get to us. So, space above our heads is mind-bendingly vast! It also means that we can, if we let ourselves, feel the enormity and specialness of witnessing the cosmos – to wonder, almost celebrate it.

We are intricately linked with the fiery furnaces in the sky that we see as stars. Most of the elements that make up our bodies, including oxygen, carbon and iron were formed in the dying throws of the cataclysmic explosions (called supernovae) of older stars through a process called stellar nucleosynthesis or nucleogenisis). This means that we are all made of stuff that was part of stars, sometimes many times over. Ultimately, the stars are where our atoms will return to so, in a way, looking to the stars is to look to our past, present and future (#Tip9 'Time Travel') literally!

If you can use binoculars or even a small telescope, there is not a patch of clear sky that doesn't have thousands of stars and other galaxies in them. It is also increasingly possible for many of us to take photographs of celestial objects. Some, like novae (the gas left after a star has exploded, or the gas around forming stars), can be very pretty and abstract in their own way (#Tip38) and are often the subject of 'space art' or 'sci-art'.

Practising being abstract and letting your mind wander when you gaze, can actually place you in a meditative state, where your brain can be calm and start noticing more of what is happening around it, as well as in it (noticing how it thinks) in less judgemental ways. This is associated with what is referred to as the brain's Default Mode Network (DMN) associated with many such reflective #Tips such as #Tip22 'Flip it' and #Tip38 'Be Abstract'.

The habit of gazing and seeing and appreciating more, is in itself a transferable skill. This has led to really fruitful collaborations between astronomers and especially medics – the skills and technologies associated with observing, processing and identifying, or diagnosing, have so much in common.

The real benefit is that this is not only a #Tip in itself but it could be the #Tip that lets you stack the most of the other #52 Tips together. Looking to the stars, usually means being outside (#Tip4, #Tip8, #Tip11, #Tip37, #Tip39), you could be listening to music (#Tip12), it allows you to breathe, wonder and consider your day (#Tip5, #Tip9, #Tip35), you can let your mind wander abstractly making connections (#Tip38) and memories (#Tip19), recalling and making stories and theories, to help reframe and contextualise your existence (#Tip9, #Tip23, #Tip47). It could become a shared pastime (#Tip34, #Tip51, #Tip52). Aside from some believing that the movement of stars and planets determines their destiny, many find the enormity of space a little scary (#Tip43).

There are also all sorts of apps that will enable you

to point a smart device to the sky to identify what you are looking at. You can set alerts and be reminded of astronomical events such as lunar eclipses, meteor showers and the passing of space stations and satellites. This can add an element of expectation and the need to 'wait for it' (#Tip37).

The sky is literally the limit with this #Tip! So next time there is a clear patch of night sky why not take a look and see what you find for yourself?

Parting Shot

This is another free #Tip that could lead to so much more, especially if you habit stack it with other #Tips. Looking to the stars may even become a passion for you if you can let yourself embrace the infinite possibilities that looking into the infinite cosmos can bring you on any clear(ish) night.

There are all sorts of online and virtual resources that you could use to get the most of looking into the night sky when you can. Even if it is cloudy, wet or just too cold, there are virtual or remote options. Many professional and amateur observatories are available online, sometimes with real time observations streamed on the internet.

This #Tip could also be renamed as: 'Make Time to Wonder' or 'Wonder it'.

41 The Best Medicine

The Big Idea

Is laughter really the best medicine? *Laughology*, so Stephanie Davies tells us in her book, is a way of seeing the world and an approach to dealing with difficulties in life. Stephanie has been really successful in taking and transitioning this concept from comedy clubs to corporate board rooms and hospital wards. It is an approach that is less about hiding or accepting difficult times and pain, but rather using humour as a way of processing and contextualising emotional experiences. Notable comedy greats that have found their calling through, and perhaps even because of, the pain they have experienced include Billy Connelly, Robin Williams and Lenny Henry.

Laughology is about learning to laugh more and to find more opportunity to do so, including laughing at ourselves. Laughter, like smiling and crying, is one of the few communication tools that is instinctive to most of us. These are universal traits, crossing cultures and borders. That said, most of us have a different sense of humour and what we find funny is not so consistent. So, how can laughter really be a top #Tip? And what makes this different from #Tip10 'Keep Smiling'?

Got it... What's the Science?

Smiling and laughing are obviously related but laughter has more of the benefits. Brain studies have shown that 'aurofacial mirror regions' (so called 'mirror neurons' that are associated with auditory processing and motor activities to do with communication), are activated in smiling, but even more so when we laugh.

Laughter is a sound we tend to make on the out-breath and we can make some very funny sounds when we do, which can make us laugh even more! Laughing is a social contagion like yawning and blinking. When we laugh genuinely, it is universally recognised by others despite any cultural background. And we tend to laugh more readily with those we know and trust, so laughter can be sign of healthy friendship and companionships.

Laughing of course can also ease tension in social situations, providing a release valve and ways out of social awkwardness, nervousness or even conflict. Laughing, appropriately in timely ways, even in difficult conversations, means that we can help others and ourselves to move on more quickly and easily, without resentment. So, the more we are prone to laughing, practising the habit and strengthening the neural wiring of laughing, by laughing more day to day, the more socially capable we can be.

What makes us laugh can be different from others and this means that laughter can be a way in which we can bond with others that see the world like ourselves and the positives this can bring – remember #Tip**34** 'Find Your Flock'. So, laughing has evolved from a basic expression of enjoyment to be a complex form of communication and is most often used in conversation by the person talking most.

Research suggests that we laugh a lot more than we think we do. Not only that, but as the use of laughter can be ambiguous, we get more savvy in working out what is meant by different types of laughter as we get older. Interestingly our brains can be more stimulated when listening to laughter that is forced or out of context. The medial prefrontal brain regions, associated with theory of mind, tend to get activated here in order to work out the context and what is really going on. Namely is it real, authentic joy-based laughter? Or forced, patronising or cynical? This processing alone hints at the complexity of laughter as a communication medium.

So, laughing is something that has a lot more going on than we first think and, on top of that, there are a number of benefits that we get immediately.

The first is biochemical. The process of laughing raises neurotransmitter levels that are uplifting in mood and sense of well-being including dopamine and serotonin. Studies have shown that those who laugh more tend to have a more optimistic view on life and are less likely to catastrophise a situation, being more able to see the opportunities from a difficult situation. Laughter also leads to the release of those natural, self-made pain-relieving neurochemicals, endorphins, that imbue us with a sense of well-being. A good hearty laugh can also be an all over body workout, involving lots of muscles and the cardiovascular system, and can lead to relaxation of muscles for up to 45 minutes afterwards. One study in Norway also suggests that those that have a strong sense of humour tend to outlive those that don't laugh as much! This effect is most notable in those battling cancer. There is also evidence that laughing actually boosts your immune system.

So, celebrate your laughter lines – you may outlive those without them!

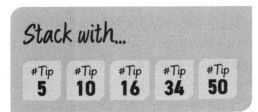

Stack with...

#Tip **5** #Tip **10** #Tip **16** #Tip **34** #Tip **50**

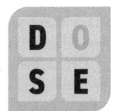

Parting Shot

You can use laughter to help you prepare to face the day. A colleague and 52 contributor, Jonathan McDonald, is in constant pain following a nasty motorcycle accident and paralysis from subsequent strokes. He daily inspires us by using radio comedies to help deal with his pain and to be able to face the night as well as day.

Repetitive inappropriate laughter can be a sign of dementia or brain damage. If you notice this in someone it might be worth suggesting that they see a doctor.

Finally, we need you to be aware that laughing more might mean you attract some people and repel others – but who do you really want to be with? And how would you prefer to see the world anyway?

#Tip 42 Make it Red

The Big Idea

When challenged to come up with a #Tip for The52Project, two executive trainees in a successful hospitality chain, Nick and Perry, came up with a simple but well-argued idea: drink a glass of red wine.

Despite having reservations about alcoholic drinks, the guys argued that there was far more to it than just a glass of wine and that, in moderation, it can be good for your health. Could this be so?

Got it... What's the Science?

This is one of those controversial science ones – with studies for and not so for this #Tip. Historically some research backs up the view that consuming a moderate amount of red wine daily, might help in the prevention of a number of conditions including heart disease. It is important to stress that this is moderate amounts, drinking one standard pub measure of 125mls – generally equivalent to one to two units of alcohol. Large glasses of 175mls are two units.

Red wines are rich in antioxidants. They come in a wide

variety of tastes and colours due to the grapes they are made from, the conditions and soil that they are grown in and the way in which they are fermented and then stored. The darker the grape, especially the skin, the more health-benefiting antioxidants such as resveratrol and proanthocyanidins they have.

Proanthocyanidins are in a group of compounds called polyphenols, that belong to a subclass called flavonoids, which give plants and berries their red, blue and purple colours. A diet that includes these compounds from fresh fruit and vegetables is known to reduce the likelihood of you getting cancer or suffering effects of ageing by lowering incidents of DNA damage.

Research shows such polyphenols can help keep your blood vessels healthy. However, research suggests an excess of extracted polyphenols may be damaging as they are without the co-benefits of plant nutrients that usually occur with a diet rich in fresh fruit and vegetables. Other studies suggest that the lowering of blood pressure is due to the relaxing effect of alcohol on our mood and therefore, only short-lived. Polyphenols may though help prevent blood clots that can cause heart attacks and strokes.

Some suggest that resveratrol (also a polyphenol) is beneficial for the healthy functioning of the central nervous system as a whole and can inhibit 'plaque' formation which is consistently associated with the neurodegenerative progression of Alzheimer's disease. People given 150 to 200mg daily resveratrol supplements have also been shown to have improved working memory or cognitive function that is thought to reflect improved cerebral blood flow (perfusion).

Other studies suggest that taking daily resveratrol as a supplement over several months may help those with type 2 diabetes by lowering glucose levels in blood as well as improving insulin resistance. BUT it should be remembered that the amount of resveratrol in a glass of wine is typically only around 1mg...

Research has also shown that moderate red wine consumption over about four weeks is associated with desirable increases in good cholesterol (HDL-C) and fibrinogen compared with drinking water with or without red grape extract. HDL-C itself is also known to be good for our health by removing excess 'bad cholesterol' (LDL-C) from blood vessels and other organs to the liver where it is broken down. HDL-C also seems to have an anti-inflammatory effect on blood vessels as well as having an antioxidant effect itself too. According to a study, the high-fibre Tempranillo red grapes, are best at lowering bad (LDL) cholesterol levels.

We can all enjoy a glass of wine at a social meal with family and friends. Arguably, moderate drinking with others can have associative psychological and well-being benefits by keeping your brain fit and healthy by stimulation and socialisation that is known to be protective against depression and the negative effects of isolation. That said, of course, alcohol is not necessary for this benefit.

Interestingly, a study by scientists from King's College London has found that red wine drinkers had a greater diversity of bacteria in their digestive tracts, a marker of gastrointestinal health, compared to those who consumed other kinds of alcohol. The suggestion here is that a greater diversity of gut bacteria means a greater ability to fight disease by being able to produce more metabolites from food. There is a plethora of research showing healthy gut flora is fundamental to healthy body functions.

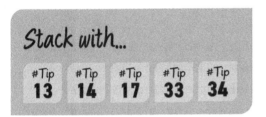

Stack with...

#Tip **13** #Tip **14** #Tip **17** #Tip **33** #Tip **34**

Parting Shot

As well as Nick and Perry, we are indebted to a list of science-based benefits compiled by Mark Davis in a blog for Whitehall Lane Winery. Moderation! Moderation! All the research conducted suggests that this is only one to two glasses (at 125mls) of red wine a day. The UK recommended weekly limit of alcohol is 14 units. Please, please, don't take this as a cue to more is better! Doctors also currently recommend having a couple of days rest from alcohol a week to give your liver a break. Alcohol is another socially acceptable, recreational drug (see #Tip**33**).

If you have had issues with keeping control of your alcohol consumption in the past, or even in your family history, please avoid this #Tip. If you are having difficulties with controlling your alcohol intake do seek medical advice from your doctor. You could also get advice from: charities such as Alcoholics Anonymous (AA) and alcoholchange.org.uk, a credible app such as MyDrinkaware App or other healthcare professionals.

Fright it

The Big Idea

Is something that frightens you necessarily bad? As you probably know the saying, a little of what scares you is good for you. To test this out we spoke with The 52 Project elite athletes, Paralympians Louise Sugden and Anna Turney, about their experiences and how it relates to performance and well-being. Both make the point that we are all either moving away from or towards our goals and fear is a valuable part of this equation.

Without challenging the fear of doing what we must to achieve what we want, the more this fear holds us back and the less likely we are to reach fulfilment. Being aware and then intentional about challenging yourself with fear can actually become exciting. Some people become addicted to the sense of achievement and confidence that they get by regularly doing this. It also seems that doing this, even a little, really helps you to become calmer when thrown out of your comfort zone – ultimately becoming more resilient.

Got it... What's the Science?

When we get scared our brain initiates a number of brain

and body processes that mean we either tend to Fight (brawl our way out of it), Flight (run away), Freeze (stop still and hope it goes away) or Flock (just do what everybody else is doing and having safety in numbers – see #Tip**34**) – the so called "4Fs". Some models also add Flop/Fatigue (for numbing or protective shutdown). These are survival strategies that we have evolved in response to threat.

Our reaction is often to give in to the fear and to avoid the uncomfortable sensations associated in attempting it. This can become a habit that serves us well enough in that we think we are safe and comfortable. The problem is that we can become risk-averse and far less capable of dealing with situations that scare us when they do happen.

The trick is not to dismiss your fear but rather to accept it without trying to fix or address it, holding off for as long as possible the Fight, Flight, Freeze or Flock reaction in situations that scare you and that you know more logically are unlikely to harm you. This is called 'urge surfing'. As we do this our heart rate slows as the brain works out that we are okay and may not be in mortal peril. As this happens more blood and oxygen are encouraged back to the PFC.

Practising this regularly means that we get used to the feeling – psychologists call it 'habituating' to the scary stimulus. For people with phobias this can be part of CBT where a client trains themselves to react more proportionately to a scary stimulus. It is important that this takes intentional effort and time and it does not have to be done alone – a professional trainer, coach or therapist can really help here.

Deliberately putting yourself out of your 'comfort

zone' into your 'stretch zone' is training. The key is not to overwhelm the body or brain and to avoid a challenge that pushes you into the 'panic zone' which would elicit the 4Fs, where brain focus is distracted from achieving the thriving (reaching or excelling in goals) by being more caught up in just surviving. Remember, at least to start with, fear of sitting with a house spider for some can be like climbing Everest or jumping out of a plane to others.

It appears that this habituation helps improve the sense of well-being thanks to serotonin messaging in the brain. Dopamine is often released after achieving a goal. So, training to overcome a challenge that scares us gives an adrenaline rush, that when accompanied by a shot of dopamine, becomes addictive. This can lead to some people becoming obsessed with the next rush that, for better or worse, translates into even more extreme activities.

It seems that a little scare regularly can give you that shot of accomplishment that can make you feel more alive day-to-day. It is likely that you will also become more confident and self-assured in your abilities generally. So, when faced with scary situations in the future you can increasingly trust yourself to come through when you really need to without hesitating or running away.

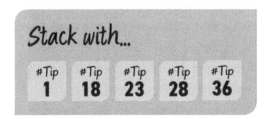

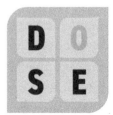

Parting Shot

Fear is an emotion that often feels irrational and that 'trumps' all other thoughts and feelings. It is very normal to be scared by specific things or contexts and not others. So choose your scare activities carefully and sensitively.

A reframe of this #Tip could be getting a bit of adventure each day which researchers in New Zealand argue is "eudaemonic" (conducive to happiness) "by supporting the satisfaction of basic psychological needs for autonomy, competence, relatedness and beneficence" (#Tip34, #Tip51). We strongly recommend caution with this #Tip. It's NOT about throwing yourself into dangerous or overwhelming situations but about regularly challenging yourself to know what it's like to feel a bit scared by being in your 'stretch zone'. If you are at all uncertain about this then do find an experienced coach or trainer. That way you will be as safe as you can be, whilst being far more likely to enjoy it and achieve that sense of accomplishment too.

If you feel scared and overwhelmed for any ongoing time, do speak to your doctor. Being constantly afraid or anxious is terrifying and unhealthy. You deserve more, so do get help with this. Online support and other help can be found at Mind (https://www.mind.org.uk) and in 'Prepare Your Personal Prescriptions'. The sooner you ask for and accept help on this, the easier your recovery will ultimately be.

Keep it

This tip from medical doctor, Dr Afiniki Akanet, is simple: have faith. As people who love science, we can sometimes give less attention to spirituality and faith, but Dr Akanet tells us why these can be good for our mental health and well-being in ways that are themselves backed by science.

We are NOT talking here about necessarily regularly attending a church, synagogue or temple or taking up religious rituals. Rather instead to intentionally see, trust and believe in the good, seen and unseen, around us. To live in and with faith in people, ourselves and / or a greater cause.

Those who have this special inner strength seem to do better mentally, even when faced with illness and other challenges. People of faith often stack several #Tips, encouraging greater mental well-being. Dr Akanet regularly makes time in her busy schedule for prayer, fasting and worship music (#Tip11, #Tip12, #Tip18, #Tip29). Her personal faith helps her to forgive others (#Tip31) and bookend her days reflecting on ancient wisdom from the Bible (#Tip35). She also enjoys laughter and hugs with friends from church (#Tip21, #Tip41), where she loves to sing and dance (#Tip16, #Tip18). Having faith, it seems, is possibly an ultimate habit stack or superstack #Tip.

Got it... What's the Science?

Paul Mueller and colleagues reported in the *Mayo Clinic Proceedings*, a prestigious peer reviewed journal of general and internal medicine, that "most studies have shown that religious involvement and spirituality are associated with better health outcomes, including greater longevity, coping skills, and health-related quality of life, even during terminal illness, and less anxiety, depression, and suicide".

Mental and physical health are, after all, naturally intimately interconnected. Poor mental and physical health then leads to a poorer quality of life and a shorter life expectancy. Many religions encourage taking better care of one's physical body by avoiding activities that have negative health consequences. So even if that is all there were to this #Tip, paying attention to one's spiritual health is worthwhile.

Having a goal focus can put you in a better, calmer place which frees up creative brain capacity and the likelihood of 'seeing' desired opportunities when they occur. Praying or meditating and believing that this will come to pass (having faith) – even without a divine intervention – could be placing our brains in the best place for those things to actually happen for us. The Bible describes faith, and puts this as, "being sure of what we hope for and certain of what we do not see," (Hebrews 11,1).

Research, from psychiatry, psychology to sociology, consistently concludes that religious people, those with an active faith, have a strong internal sense of control. People with a so-called 'healthy faith' (that is not a cultist or fundamentalist faith) also feel in control of their free will to believe or not to believe, thereby choosing the beliefs that guide their actions.

Socio-psychological models that, like Gregory Bateson and Robert Dilts' (neuro)logical levels, extol well-being and fulfilment do so by means of so called 'aligning' lives with environments, behaviours, values with identity and some ultimately a faith, or greater good, at its pinnacle.

Unfortunately, faith can come with some downsides too. It's sadly not uncommon for people to suffer and hold themselves in anxiety or depression, even captive, to thoughts of a vengeful deity, being "punished by God" – or indeed punishing others for a different faith, doctrine or practice. Perhaps a shadow side of the tribal drive we have seen in #Tip34 'Find Your Flock'.

These can of course be extremely harmful and should be mindfully guarded against. Fundamentalism or fatalism in any belief, organisation or system is limiting and counterproductive to a fuller and respect of, and for, life with ourselves and others – especially if it leads to violence, intolerance or discrimination.

Like art, spirituality and religions can however also offer a deeper hope and purpose to difficult, existential questions that medical professionals and scientists cannot as easily help us with – like: what is the meaning of my life?

It is recognised that good medical consultations include an exploration of a patient's spirituality and beliefs as part of a more holistic approach to their healthcare. Arguably this includes patient trust and faith in the clinicians as well as the science and the medical basis for treatments used. So, in many ways, faith and beliefs are very much part of patient care – dare we say science too?

An interesting 2019 article in *Forbes* by Nicole Roberts explains: "Compassion, forgiveness and gratefulness are also qualities that are strongly associated with individuals who are spiritual and religious. Practising these qualities is thought to be associated with decreased stress and increased resilience".

If this is not enough, a study of just over 1,500 obituaries across the US by scientists in Ohio State University concluded that those that were 'religiously affiliated' lived between five and a half and nine and three-quarter years longer than those who didn't.

Stack with
#Tips
**3, 12, 16, 18, 21, 26, 29, 31,
34, 35, 38, 40, 41, 45, 47, 51, 52**

Parting Shot

This is a tip that could also help with finding your flock (#Tip34), that might unlock connectedness, hope, optimism, trust and purpose. If you already have a particular faith, it might be worthwhile reconnecting with a positive, helpful like-minded belief-based community, and forming daily habits that help you stay healthy and live purposefully. We are not saying who or what here – we are simply recognising the science and wisdom of having and keeping a faith!

Trust it

The Big Idea

When it comes to making decisions, many of us will have a 'gut feel' about what is the best choice under the circumstances. Sometimes, however, we don't want to trust ourselves to decide without some 'proper facts' to back up our gut feel. Instead of getting on with something, we might check out what data there is, or we might put off deciding by telling ourselves it is sensible and grown up to do some research first so that we don't make a mistake.

This data might give us a sense that our decision is more likely to be right, but is that true? Does being furnished with more facts necessarily make our decision a better one?

Sometimes there is nothing better than just going with your instincts, because actually making decisions based on your emotions turns out to be much more reliable than you might imagine.

Got it... What's the Science?

Malcolm Gladwell's international bestseller, *Blink – The Power of Thinking without Thinking*, is all about the phenomenon of how snap judgements can be far more effective than our more cautious calculated decisions – how a firefighter suddenly 'feels' he must get out of a building, or someone on a speed date just 'knows' that this is the right one.

In Cordelia Fine's book, *A Mind of Its Own*, there is a wealth of psychological experiments to pick from that help us learn all sorts of things about our brains.

The one that we think helps most here is a gambling game played with a deck of cards meant to simulate real-life decision making, called the 'IOWA Gambling Task'. Players were asked to select cards over and over again from four different decks in front of them. Drawing particular cards would win them or lose them points. Two of the decks had some big wins in them. but also some big losses that were best avoided. The other two decks were better in the long run – the wins weren't as big but neither were the losses.

In this experiment the players eventually realised that the more moderate decks were the 'best packs' – they had that 'aha' moment when they realised what was going on. And most of them had developed a 'hunch' that one deck was better than the other before they were conscious of it and had started to select more cards from it.

As well as being observed, the participants in the study were also monitored by skin conductance equipment which uses electricity to measure sweat. This showed that long before any of the participants had their 'aha' moment, and even before they were showing any inclination to follow a 'hunch', their sweat glands knew already! That is, subconsciously, their brains were autonomically setting their body up. Just before they were about to touch a card from the risky deck, they would have an emotional jolt which they couldn't feel but which showed up on the sweat monitors. Only after those 'invisible' emotional jolts were repeated a few times did the 'gut feel' kick in.

This experiment helps us to understand that gut feel is not luck or coincidence and doesn't just come from nowhere. It comes from the combined functions of the brain that process emotions, senses and predicts patterns and perceives 'wholeness'. This lets the more logical, rational and conscious giving parts of our brain know that something is going on and that we should start paying attention to it!

The interesting thing is where we sense this feeling or source here. All sensations are perceived in the brain but we feel them in our gut. It helps to think of the nervous system as a whole system and this 'referred' sensation is called somatisation.

Functional MRI (fMRI) brain scan studies have also looked for centres where this processing is occurring. Brain regions that 'light up' when intuition is being 'prompted' include the medial parietal cortex and the right superior temporal cortex. These regions of the brain have been associated with a sense of self and wholeness as well as sensing when something is deviating from the whole or normal.

It seems that the more experience you have in doing something, the more likely your brain will subconsciously know when something feels right or not. So, when you do go with your intuition, far from just plucking something from the air, it's your brain as alerted by your whole nervous system.

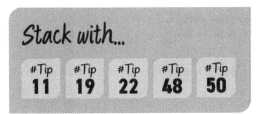

Stack with...

#Tip	#Tip	#Tip	#Tip	#Tip
11	19	22	48	50

Parting Shot

The more positive feedback we get by going with our intuition, the better and more confident we are at 'hearing', 'listening' and going with it. Dr Dan Harrison, in his balance of behavioural paradoxes for making decisions, has a graph where the y-axis is being analytical (logical) and the x-axis is going with intuition (non-logical). According to Harrison, making excellent decisions involves 'balanced versatility' in both the extremes of 'x' and 'y': the top-right of the graph, a zone called 'logical intuition'. This is a particularly valuable leadership trait.

So, a key to a better, and a more 'top-right' type of thinking, capable of better resolving challenges and problems, especially in the moment, is using more of your brain, more of the time: using both the conscious logical and the intuitive non-logical processing. This is a concept that is extended in Daniel Kahneman's book, *Thinking Fast and Slow*.

If you want better intuition, the more exposure and deliberate practice you can give your brain, the more likely it will prove useful for you – even if, at first, you don't know why...

#Tip 46 Perfectly Imperfect

The Big Idea

They say that beauty is in the eye of the beholder. For something to be truly beautiful it probably has to be imperfect. In a world where celebrities and products are celebrated for being ever more perfect do we also place a huge and, ultimately, self-defeating expectation on ourselves and others?

Body dysmorphia, where sufferers are racked with anxiety about a physical defect that others don't seem to see, is a mental health condition – what we 'see', we perceive and what we perceive we 'see' as real. Perception is influenced by our paradigms and schemas (#Tip9, #Tip19, #Tip22, #Tip23, #Tip31, #Tip47). We have been socially conditioned to think what is beautiful.

Across Europe and the USA it is estimated that roughly one in fifty people suffer from body dysmorphia disorder (BDD). That means that there are tens of millions of people who don't think that they are normal, let alone beautiful, with all the pain, separation and rejection that this causes. The increasing pressures that social media places particularly on young people are likely to make this sobering statistic even worse in the future.

So, is there anything we can do about it? Can we start to

see beauty and value in other ways, even in the imperfect?

In traditional Japanese aesthetics, *Wabi Sabi*, is a view that something is accepted, even valued, because of its imperfections or short livedness' (transience). *Kintsugi* is similarly where broken things are revered by being restored with precious metals, celebrating their history. In this #Tip we are borrowing again from ancient wisdom, so that we may learn to accept ourselves more; to enjoy and value ourselves and help others to do the same; to both release and empower us through finding strength from our life stories, rather than hiding the imperfect and broken pieces.

Got it... What's the Science?

There are some facial features that our brains seem to take particular interest in when looking at other faces. We tend to be attracted to faces that have eyes that are identically as far apart as our own. We also tend to trust faces and smiles if they are 'dynamically symmetrical' (#Tip10).

The pursuit of perfection or at least attraction to ideals of self is almost as old as animal-kind itself. Certain features are believed to represent greater likelihood of reproductive success and status symbols, like larger antlers, vibrant colours or more external aesthetics like well-ordered nests. These become the things that are the desired or 'beautiful' traits. Most organisms seek to be more like these and if they are not naturally endowed, there can be considerable efforts made to make up for this. Makeup, used since at least ancient

Egyptian eras, is meant to cover up blemishes and highlight features associated with beauty and desired traits.

We are humbled by those who have shared their stories with us, especially around disfigurement from birth, or accident, as well as those who suffer from BDD. Their journeys have inspired us to strive to find an internal strength and a kind of inside out beauty from the things that have left their mark on us. This includes both mental and physical scars. In a touching scene in the 80s film *Shirley Valentine*, Shirley's admirer and lover Costas kisses her stretch marks and says "they are lovely, because they are part of you, and you are lovely, so don't hide, be proud. They are the marks of life."

This acceptance of differences and imperfections can of course be much easier said than done for ourselves. However, rather than being a source of shame and trying to hide them, our perceived imperfections can provide assurance and an earned inner strength. Michael Phelps's body features of unusually large palms and feet, short legs and long body, have arguably made him more beautiful and faster in the water – his differences helped to make him the most decorated Olympian to date. Ongoing success for Michael, both literal and mental, has come from a self-acceptance that includes not just seeing the elite swimmer in the mirror. Undoubtedly this also came with hard fought reframing in his mind of who he is, which would be confirmed by the story he told himself (see #Tip**23**). The voice our brain listens to most often is our own – this is our greatest challenge with this #Tip and subject of our next #Tip.

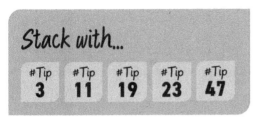

Stack with...

#Tip	#Tip	#Tip	#Tip	#Tip
3	**11**	**19**	**23**	**47**

Parting Shot

What flaws or scars, both visible and invisible, do you feel you have? How could you at least start to celebrate these as part of you being you and your journey? And if you did, how could these be used for a force for good for you and others?

We are not saying we all have to just accept or settle for our own perceived flaws and imperfections, after all this is a big part of why we strive to improve ourselves and get better at habits by practising and stacking them, but maybe there is more to life if we can embrace the asymmetric, quirky and unusual rather than seeking to keep them hidden.

Winning at this is actually to be brave and seek support and help, rather than hide from it. This is another #Tip you don't need to do by yourself. Who do you know and trust who could help you with this? Don't forget there is professional help available if you seek it.

Last thought, stamps and coins are more valuable to collectors if they have errors or mistakes. Just saying!

#Tip 47 **Speak it Out**

The Big Idea

If you are regularly told by someone close, "You will never be able to do that!" or, "You look terrible," you'd be really affronted and probably try to spend less time around them. So, what happens when that negative, overly critical voice is coming from YOU?

Many of us speak to ourselves every day with an inner dialogue called 'self-talk', which we barely notice unless we deliberately pay attention to who it is. Research suggests that most of our self-talk about ourselves is negative. The National Science Foundation (USA) reportedly published an article in 2005 that proposed that most of us have about 12,000 to 60,000 thoughts each day, of which about 80% are negative. What's more, as much as 95% are the same repetitive thoughts as the day before. It seems your mind, left to its own devices, gets stuck in a negative self-talk loop which is keeping you down.

But there is an alternative. Our friend, Gabor Kocsi, has been practising positive affirmations every day for years and has great personal stories that this simple #Tip really makes a BIG difference to himself and others around him.

Actively choosing to tell ourselves something positive in the morning, reflecting on the positive things we have done, and then creating an associated affirmation such as "I add value to the lives of the people around me" doesn't just make us feel better in the moment, it actually becomes true. And the more you use it, the more it becomes true.

Gabor reminded us that what we say to ourselves can have a huge impact on how we feel and act and therefore, every day we can have a choice and authority over how we turn up to work and live our lives.

Got it... What's the Science?

Our perception of our own world, the metaphoric lenses, 'paradigms' and cognitive biases, through which we view that world, together with our patterns of thinking, or 'schemas' (#Tip9, #Tip19, #Tip22, #Tip23), are all influenced by the language that we and others use on ourselves.

Saying something positive means that your brain is much more likely to look for opportunities for that positive thing to happen and find evidence that the positive thing is already true. The problem with the brain is that all too often the reverse is true. We tell ourselves something negative which we didn't really witness and away in the background our brain gets busy looking for evidence that the negative thing is true and finds opportunities to confirm it. This is another shadow side to 'confirmation bias' (#Tip3, #Tip22), one of well over 150 characterised cognitive biases, which all interfere with how we process signals and information, think critically, and perceive reality.

The negative self-talk we use is most likely related to, and fuel for, 'imposter syndrome' which, some researchers suggest affects at least 70% of us at some point in our lives. The positive intent of this pattern of thinking is to try and help keep you safe, but it can also stop you really living.

Flipping this pattern is like trying to flip the life-long habit of seeing a glass half-empty to seeing it half-full. It takes effort. Even if you are a glass half full thinker, there is likely room for improvement to make it more so. This takes awareness, intent, deliberate practice and time, which is where positive words and affirmations help to more positively shape your reality and possibility.

A brain scanning (fMRI) study published in 2016 has given early indicators of the neural circuits and brain regions that are thought to be involved with these self-affirmation tasks. The authors of this paper pointed to the roles of the Ventral Striatum (VS) and Ventral Medial Prefrontal Cortex (VMPFC), regions associated with expectation and receipt of positively valued or rewarding outcomes. The authors went on to highlight the connection between VMPFC activity in imagining positive future events, which may be significant in the way positive affirmations 'play forwards' to affect processing towards a goal, raising the likelihood that you will make internal aspirations a perceived as well as 'real' reality. The study, along with a bit of logic, suggest that the more thought out the goals of the affirmation are, the more likely they are to have the desired impact.

Coaches know that the greater the clarity of the goal, the greater the impact and likelihood of promoting the outcome.

Too many words of affirmation or too many reasons, are likely to dilute the impact. We suggest finding and regularly using short phrases or sayings that resonate with your well-defined, desired purpose and core values are most likely to give you the impact you want. When you get evidence that this is working, you will gain even more confidence that you are on the right track for you, which will in turn give you a greater sense of purpose in this process. This is your brain consolidating the wiring for your success. It all starts by you challenging the negative self-talk you use about yourself.

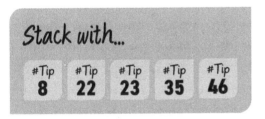

Stack with...

#Tip	#Tip	#Tip	#Tip	#Tip
8	**22**	**23**	**35**	**46**

Parting Shot

When you deliberately form optimistic thought patterns and see setbacks as temporary this will become your default setting – a 'growth mindset' (**#Tip8**, **#Tip32**). You can become a 'mood radiator' (see **#Tip28**) that people want to be around, a beacon of positivity and a leader that doesn't have to be pushy to realise their dreams – like our friend Gabor.

How about writing down, or even doodling, your positive affirmations on post-it notes and sticking them somewhere that you will see regularly, like the fridge door, a mirror, or computer screen?

Slow it Down

The Big Idea

We all know that yoga is associated with wellness and meditation. The ancient practice originated in India as a group of physical, mental and spiritual practices aimed at stilling the mind. In more recent times, in the Western world, it has become a posture-based fitness, stress-relief and relaxation technique found on apps and on YouTube videos.

It seems fairly obvious that frequent yoga will be beneficial for you physically, by toning and strengthening your muscles, whilst increasing your flexibility. However, most of us don't really appreciate the reasons why it is so beneficial for us beyond that. It isn't just a bit of stretching and breathing, it also has many mental and cognitive benefits that we can use every day, in the moment, beyond the yoga mat.

Got it... What's the Science?

Multiple studies have shown that practices used in yoga can decrease the secretion of cortisol, as well as bring on the sense of calm that is associated with increasing 'vagal tone' associated with breathing (#Tip**5**). When we explored

#Tip**5** it was apparent that breathing is very under-valued and all too often something that we do poorly – most of the time. Being more deliberate and practised with breathing, especially when pulling some moves, means we are also practising for when breathing is more difficult in, say, stressful situations.

Practising means that the pathways and confidence in the techniques become a lot easier to actually do when we most need them. By increasing breathing and oxygen to the PFC, we are also making creative thinking more possible. This can mean that when we come to slowing things down, to smooth them out, we can do them faster and, therefore, better. Slower means noticing, being more fluid, more creative, more in control, more able to see the wood for the trees – especially when under pressure. The US Navy Seals famously have a mantra: "slow is smooth, smooth is fast" – for this very reason. By the way, using breath control is useful in all sorts of life activities from freediving to getting to sleep (#Tip**24**).

By deliberately focusing on body areas, in yoga and similar and associated disciplines like Pilates and meditation, we become more aware of them. This can sometimes manifest in us feeling the warmth of energy 'flow' into and through our bodies. From a science point of view this perception is probably brought about by the bioelectric activity of our nervous system. Others would argue that there is more 'tuning in' to the universe or universal energies. In #Tip**39** we also referenced that 'grounding' may well have its 'scientific' place here too. We are, after all, bioelectric beings interacting with other physical energies – in energy terms, none of us is an island.

One of the other great benefits activities such as yoga and Pilates gives most of us is exercise with a low risk of injuring muscles and ligaments. By balancing activity of opposing muscle groups, in a non-competitive, process-oriented activity we can start to open up almost limitless possibilities for growth in self-awareness. It is this practice of balancing opposing forces that arguably helps us recognise and so gain better balance in our lives off the yoga mat too.

The amazing multitude of stretch and 'mechano' receptors in our bodies helps us become even more aware of a body-map that we have in our brains. If you were to draw a line connecting your ears over the top of your head, this map sits towards the upper surface of your brain, just behind this central line on both sides of your head (just behind and along the central gyrus in the parietal lobes) and is called the primary somatosensory cortex (S1). Research from minute electrical stimulation of human brains by scientists published by Wilder Penfield and Edwin Boldly back in 1937, led to this map being represented as a homunculus (a 3D human statue), where body parts were sized proportionate to their alleged sensitivity – called Penfield's Homunculus. This map or homunculus is constantly being 'accessed', added to, and maintained each and every day which means it is both a living map and 'plastic' as in neuroplastic. If you have a limb amputated then this is reflected by a change in the map. This electrical stimulating process is still used by neurosurgeons, like Rahul Jandial, as they map areas to avoid when surgically removing tumours from the brain, so as to avoid damaging areas particularly to do with movement and language.

Combined, the meditation aspect of yoga, breathing (#Tip5), mindfulness and concentration can all help you to exercise and strengthen key connections (synapses) - 'wiring' and 'circuitry' in your brain so that you are more capable of in the moment of going slow, to go fast, and to be resilient. To not only survive but to thrive through life's pressures and storms.

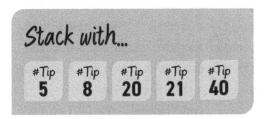

Stack with...

| #Tip 5 | #Tip 8 | #Tip 20 | #Tip 21 | #Tip 40 |

Parting Shot

The bottom line is that multiple studies have confirmed the many mental and physical benefits of yoga, and by incorporating it into your routine it can help enhance your health, increase your strength and flexibility and even reduce symptoms of stress, depression and anxiety. Finding the time to add yoga to your routine just a few times a week should be enough to make a noticeable difference to your well-being. Yet another example where science is catching up with and reflecting ancient wisdom.

Joy of Missing Out (JOMO)

The Big Idea

Most of us have heard of FOMO, the Fear of Missing Out. It's been fuelled by social media and the wizardry of algorithms tailoring the advertising we receive. We're conditioned to think that by not doing / having / going to / achieving something, we're going to miss out. In everyday life, you might miss an in-joke, an opportunity or being 'seen', and if you don't do or buy it, you should be really fearful because something is wrong – worse, you could be wrong.

This is a social hang-up that probably exists to make sure we stay as a tribe, which has helped us survive as a species. And fear is not necessarily a bad thing. We know from #Tip43 that occasionally being a bit scared can be good for us. That said, we also know that fear can also close down the PFC and so creative thinking, options and even awareness. Repetitive or protracted periods of fear can certainly be debilitating and destructive to our well-being, self-confidence and sense of self.

In this #Tip, Jen (AKA Digital Jen), challenges us to flip this narrative: to think what we could get, or actually be saying yes to, if we could get better at saying no to, and miss out on, others. So rather than losing out, what could we gain? Could there actually be such a thing as JOMO – a Joy of Missing Out?

Got it... What's the Science?

FOMO is what psychologists, sociologists and anthropologists would call a form of 'social conditioning', a kind of 'group think' (another bias), to help us as families or groups to conform, to be cohesive and stay together. Being fearful of not joining in is really to be afraid of the social consequences which can impact our status or standing within a social group. Missing out means we don't keep up, making it harder to catch up what might have been. By being 'fearful' of this means we are less likely to miss out on whatever the 'it' is that everyone else is doing.

Arguably, FOMO can incentivise us, because it is about what possibilities are out there for people like us. Unfortunately, with the privilege of so many possibilities, we can end up snatching at all sorts of opportunities that might lead to even more possibilities and opportunities, which can give even more FOMO. We can become increasingly fearful that we might miss THE one that really makes the difference. It all gets jumbled up, leaving us feeling exhausted, confused, uncertain and fearful, and actually less well off than before. We call this state 'FOMO-lock' or 'FOMO-block'; struggling to know what we really want or who we really are. Increasingly, this is being recognised as a psychological condition that doctors, therapists, and psychologists are becoming concerned about.

By losing the connection and the associated dopamine and oxytocin hits, or confusing the signals, we can lose touch and control of how to predict what these possibilities can give us and why we need them in the first place. In effect we start losing touch with reality the more that we are 'plugged in' to all of the options, all of the time. Our brains' 'hardware' and social 'programming', is not built for going at a such relentless pace, with so many twists and turns of 'shoulds'. FOMO can all too easily be a slippery slope into chronic fearful uncertainty, anxiety and depression, even self-loathing. The FOMO ultimately means we are more likely to miss out!

So, what's the answer?

As in so many ancient wisdoms it's simply to simplify. Less is indeed more. In our experience, this is easier said than done. For those of us who get energy from connection and validation from others, or even things, it can be a deeper trap than we might think.

So we suggest that by flipping the FOMO to JOMO you can actually get a dopamine hit from being yourself and for choosing to live with the discomfort of missing out, instead focusing this fear energy into what you are doing in the moment. Like a Jedi, the real power of our present is in how it determines our destiny (#Tip8). By choosing less you can actually be getting more. Next time you are feeling a FOMO try this instead: slow down (#Tip48), breathe (#Tip5), maybe reframe the situation (#Tip23) and notice the small moments and the things that are before you (#Tip8, #Tip11). In doing so, you are much more likely to be with the people (flock/s) that really matter to you (#Tip34). Deliberately practising and exercising JOMO can be really empowering, even enjoyable. We believe JOMO can unlock being the master of your own destiny rather than at the whim of others'.

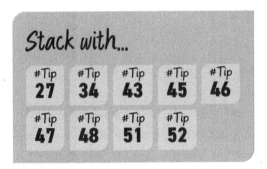

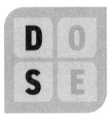

Parting Shot

This might not be one that you want to try but we suggest it is probably one that you need. This #Tip will require a bit of bravery and maybe letting some stuff, even relationships, go **#Tip31**. It might also mean disconnecting, to wake up to the opportunities that are already at your feet or right in front of you. Remember, "where the attention goes, the energy flows." JOMO means you can be more ready to be and do what you want and need to. And so to be ultimately happier.

#Tip 50 Play

The Big Idea

Play or die! When you stop making connections and learning new things, your brain actually starts to die. Some would even say that when you stop enjoying life, you start to 'lose' in the 'game of life'.

Amongst ourselves we were surprised and a little embarrassed at how, even though we think of ourselves as fun, we have got out of the habit of playing. There are those that play sport but that's sport, and sport is often serious and generally competitive. Play is different. Play is not efficient, it doesn't tend to have hard and fast rules, and it can feel frivolous, only to be entertained with our children or when the 'real' work has been done.

Many mammals play as a part of their everyday lives. Nature doesn't keep things by accident so, if play has remained in evolutionary terms, then surely there's some good reasons for it. And if that's true, are we 'grown-ups' missing something that most of us found, literally, child's play when we were children? This is a #Tip we have been inspired to explore thanks to Sara Sibai, who elevates and energises leaders and teams all over the world through the power of play. According to Sara, missing play literally means missing out on life.

Got it... What's the Science?

When we play, we enact situations that could be useful for us. In animals this is often to prepare for survival, being independent or part of a team. When we get enjoyment from activities we get a dopamine boost, especially if we surprise ourselves by doing better, find out or achieve more than we thought that we would. Play also involves a degree of physical activity which helps with our fitness, loosening us up as well as releasing tension which then leads to the release of euphoric endorphins (#Tip20).

As children, we let ourselves inhabit the imaginary in a way that we tend to close off as adults. The proportion of random neuronal connections in the brain is greater when we are children. This means that we can encode situations and our responses more diversely as children. Our brains are more 'fluid' and adaptive, or 'plastic', when young. Part of the role of the PFC is to inhibit inappropriate behaviour. This is less developed in children so there is less tendency to be inhibited or judge in the way an adult might. This predisposes younger children to play and share in play with each other.

The Nobel Prize winning physiologist and medic, Gerald Eldelman, proposed a model of neural evolution involving brain architecture and 'wiring', where associations that are positive or useful are strengthened and retained and where those that aren't or don't, 'wither' to insignificance or ineffectiveness. In theory, the more we practised and the more diverse our play was as a child, the more we retain the architecture to make broader, creative connections later in life. As we move into adulthood we go through a period of significant 'neural' or 'synaptic' pruning. This means we tend to swap creativity and plasticity for efficiency and speed in processing.

This is an evolutionary survival technique – quick reactions used to be the difference between life and death. In terms of our selfish gene(s), as Prof. Richard Dawkins would put it, the objective is for us to pass on characteristics and experience that historically imbues quick, appropriate reactions, whilst having offspring who can also retain the ability to see and do things more creatively in case the 'game of life' changes in the meantime. This phenomenon brings a balance between individual growth and corporate social evolution as a species.

As adults we can still play! Like a muscle, the more we practice making random mental connections and associations the more likely we are to keep and strengthen our abilities to be creative and flexible (#Tip**38**). Humour is important here too (#Tip**41**). Shared humour allows us to 'play' together with metaphors and concepts, whilst, temporarily, not needing to get it right. This is rocket fuel to a growth mindset and to those that seek to lead themselves and others in such a Volatile, Uncertain, Complex and Ambiguous (VUCA) world. Because, to paraphrase Einstein, "the thinking that has got us here, will need to be different to get us there..." – where 'there' is better than here.

Experiences that have shaped how we think come from a limited lifetime of experience. Play can change this, releasing and realising an 'extended mind', by unlocking other perspectives in the ways you and your fellow players, can 'see' and envision – to individually as well as corporately experience through imagination. Dr James Carse characterised these types of games as 'Infinite Games' where you invite many other players along the way and keep playing the game. In contrast, 'Finite Games' limit the number of players and the outcomes to winners and losers.

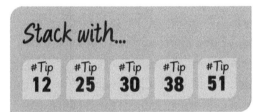

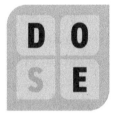

Parting Shot

Play helps you to remain young, literally, and can connect across generations in a way other types of communication don't. It is even thought that being playful helps you live longer.

Play is also such an important part of the innovation process that inventors and entrepreneurs such as Sir James Dyson introduced a monthly play day for staff, where employees can literally play in other departments – for the sake of just seeing what they can do and make together. Play, after all, is arguably the purest fuel to innovation and possibility.

#Tip
51 Offer it

The Big Idea

The gifts we value most are the ones that are thought through and personal, where we feel someone really understands us. Similarly, most of us get satisfaction from giving gifts that shows the recipient that we have thought about them considerately too.

Receiving gifts is one of Gary Chapman's *Five Love Languages* and involves degrees of emotional intelligence.

Giving of these 'languages' is a two-way process, with emotional and sometimes physical benefits to receivers and givers. This is different to RAK (**#Tip26**), because it is about stoking the fires for closer relationships and so is a far more involved, ongoing process. This #Tip requires it to be an invitation where an offer can, and should, be possible to turn down. In contrast, our RAKs are generally defined as one-way actions with little or no ongoing close interactions.

What you are offering, like a lift or something to eat, may seem fairly trivial. The key is in the intention. The process of building on emotional intelligence to deepen relationships with others, means the receiver remains in control of whether to receive it or not. This usually amplifies the impact of the offer and so deepens the relationship of mutual trust and respect much further (**#Tip34**).

Got it... What's the Science?

We have centres and cells in our brains that 'mirror' the actions of others as if we were doing them, but at a much lower level of activation or excitement – below the threshold for actual physical movement. These have been coined 'mirror neurons'. Their actual existence remains controversial, but as conceptual entities they allow us to copy and learn by imitating others and are probably involved in helping us to decipher the intention of others. Mirror neurons enable us to reflect others' facial expressions, actions, body language and emotions and to reproduce them.

The observation of others activates our mirror neurons which means we start using our brain wiring to live out what another person is doing and going through, especially if we are invested in that person or their actions. This is used regularly in army and healthcare services training, where individuals are 'drilled' with a maxim of 'watch one, do one, teach one' or 'watch, imitate, demonstrate' to help acquire, learn and pass on best practice.

Simply learning these responses allows even those with high functioning autism to learn appropriate responses to others' emotions or behaviour. It is the emotional link and exchange that can be harder, to convert or feel, for those with autism.

When we make the link to what someone else is doing, and we are invested in a relationship with that person, oxytocin is involved. An EEG study published in 2010 by Prof. Richard Ebstein and others suggests that oxytocin can help activate the mirror neuron system/s. As such, oxytocin may be a therapeutic approach for those with autism.

When we are valued, we receive a 'virtual hug' (#Tip21). In Transactional Analysis terms these are called 'pats' and 'strokes' and are meta-physical or metaphoric, not actual. The suggestion is that we need a sufficient number of 'pats' and 'strokes' a day to survive, let alone thrive. This could be why isolation can be so difficult for many of us and why solitary confinement is used as a form of torture. In offering an action that validates and supports another, we mirror this hug ourselves and receive the immediate benefits. The more apt the offer of help, the greater this hit is likely to be for both parties and the greater the relational benefits that result.

It is important that the offer is a genuine exchange that can be turned down by the person you are trying to help. If an offer becomes a demand, we provoke a threat response from that person. This makes the person feel under-valued and more wary of you in the future. In David Rock's SCARF model, 'A' stands for Autonomy, having control and ownership of one's own actions. Those with a love language of 'receiving gifts', can struggle to see why someone else wouldn't want their offer and so end up offering it more forcefully. If we don't allow someone to turn down our offer, we weaken the very relationship we are trying to build.

So, 'mirroring' is important for both offerors and receivers (offerees) – being a foundation in building and maintaining healthy relationships, self-esteem and even status, in our social groups. The more you practise the habit of 'offering', the more you exercise your emotional intelligence brain circuits. With the greater feedback you will get from regular receivers, you will improve your social and emotional intelligence and capabilities – all with the very welcome added benefit of feeling valued, even loved, as part of the same process!

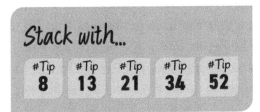

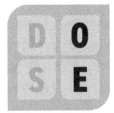

Parting Shot

Be genuine with what you offer. You need to be invested enough to follow through with your offer to help in the way that you said that you would and which has been mutually agreed upon.

Don't overcommit. Try to be realistic with what you offer and when, or you will undermine the intention to help if you can't honour it.

Be prepared for your offer to be respectfully turned down. Insisting that someone accepts your offer makes it a demand. Make it OK for someone to say, "no, thank you."

#Tip
52 Pass it On

The Big Idea

As we come to the last #Tip, we are mindful that if you have learnt something that you have put into practice to change your life for the better, one of the best things you can do for yourself, and others, is to now Pass it On.

This #Tip builds so much on the #Tips and habits that we have been working on throughout this book and it's a #Tip that naturally stacks with any other #Tip!

And the process of passing it on, as in advice, as a gift, as an offer (#Tip51), means that we are far more likely to take action on that advice ourselves and, in so doing, change our lives and our world for the better.

Got it... What's the Science?

Throughout this book we have touched on some of the neurochemicals that support us in our relationships. We often feel better when we have given something of value to others and by giving gifts, the neurochemicals of 'happiness' here include the interplay of the now hopefully familiar trifecta of dopamine, serotonin and oxytocin.

But the benefits of these chemicals don't stop at happiness

or a sense of well-being. We have spoken about how healthier balances of these chemicals in your life can help to decrease stress, reduce inflammation and chronic illness, improve sleep and memory, promote a healthier appetite and even raise your confidence and sex-drive - each of which generally lead to increased opportunities for happiness.

The passing on of what we have learnt is a way in which we can illicit similar responses in others so that everyone benefits (#Tip26, #Tip51).

Occasionally we can get the idea that we are in competition with other people. It can feel self-empowering to hold on to a 'secret' to health, wealth and happiness because it gives you a perceived edge on those around you, like you are getting ahead of the pack. This is probably a hang up from the need for competition to drive survival both at the individual and species level.

When we do compete and look out for number one, it is usually because of some shaky belief that this will make us more successful and better, even better to help others. But offering and giving the gift of considerate help and support (#Tip51) and sharing experiences and stories, thereby passing on #Tips that have helped us, means that you can be more effective as a friend, colleague or partner.

A small Italian study published in 2019, involving couples exchanging gifts at the beginning or partway through a gaming task, explored the link between gift exchange, gratitude and cognitive effects. Results showed a correlation between gift giving and improvements in game performance that they associated with increased neural activity in the dorsal lateral prefrontal cortex (DLPFC). This region is concerned with how to react to stimuli and other 'executive' functions such as cognitive flexibility, planning, abstract reasoning and inhibition of inappropriate behaviour. The study's authors suggest that the improvement in co-operative game performance is the result of triggered empathetic attitudes that function to give positive feedback for promoting pro-social behaviour and interaction. The giving and receiving of gifts made them think that they were more connected and 'on-board' with the task at hand, which, ultimately, meant that they were, and everyone 'won' / benefitted (see #Tip**50**).

Passing on a #Tip means you both benefit in being better together – as the researchers put it, "receiving but also donating is related to an enhancement of cooperative bonds." This is another example of one of our favourite Andrew Jenkins' quotes: "I to the power of we" – as in maths: I^{we}. When I 'win' you 'win', when you and I 'win', we 'win', which means I 'win' and so on. Importantly, this is a power function, so that the result is exponentially greater than the addition.

When giving advice we need to be careful not to be judgemental or overly persistent and the #Tip has to be an offer so as not to provoke a threat response, that would be counter-productive (#Tip**51**).

Research published in 2018 by researchers at the University of Pennsylvania and University of Chicago, suggests that giving advice or passing on a #Tip can actually be more beneficial than receiving it. Their research showed that after an experiment, 72% of people were motivated to action by / through giving advice in the experiment, compared to just 34% before the experiment. It is likely that the process of thinking why a #Tip would be useful to someone else means that you think it through more thoroughly for yourself, making it more relevant to your situation. So, whether the person you share the #Tip with takes it or not, by thinking it out to share it, you get the increased motivation and foresight to make it actually happen – and so you get the #Tip benefits for yourself!

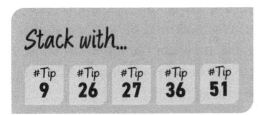

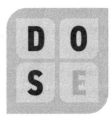

Parting Shot

As Yoda says: "pass on what you have learned." This is one of the very best habit-stacks that you can do. By being ready to offer a #Tip to those you think would benefit from it, you have a mindset of abundance over scarcity. Research has shown that abundant givers, who understand and value what they are giving, are the greatest 'winners' in life.

Think of someone that matters to you in your team or family. What one #Tip do you think would help them? What one #Tip have you found most useful in the last year? Pass it on and see what it can do for you and them.

And That's it, Folks!

Parting Shot

That's it. 52 tips for a happier life and the science to back them, and you, up. Remember you can use these anytime and make more of them by combining or 'stacking' them. As with all interventions, it's about finding a balance of what works for you. Together these can form your own personal prescription to a happier life.

We hope that you will agree that the #Tips all meet our five criteria for inclusion in this project and so this book:

1) Easy to do
2) Accessible (or adaptable) for almost anyone
3) Cheap or free
4) Stackable with other tips
5) Have definite scientific back-up.

The 52 Project isn't over, it continues with you! To help you further do visit our blogs and website at The52Project. com. We will add more #Tips as we come across them, so please share any of your favourite tips that we are missing – or feel free to ask us to science-check a new one that you come across!

Don't forget you can read more, find more links and videos, as well as access references and sources to all the #Tips at: https://the52project.com

You can still watch the 52Tips that we recorded live @52Tips on Instagram. Join our community by following us and let's all share more of what we know and find out about feeling happier, living well and getting more out of life. We would love to hear your stories and where you take this, your own project, next.

A Note on DOSE

So there I (Iain) was on a dog walk in the middle of a wood, lost, at dusk, when Dulcie called me posing the idea of using DOSE (Dopamine – Oxytocin – Serotonin – Endorphin) as a self-styled, self-help pharmaceutical palette. The more we talked, the more merit and credence we could see in it as a useful model to help others. My dog and I found the path out of the wood and Dulcie's mind continued to work on producing the 4-quadrant palette. This pairing of thoughts and discussions that were foundational in what has become The52Project and this book.

There are two important aspects that we would like to acknowledge here.

Firstly, it turns out, like many an idea, that others have also found and used DOSE as a useful model. Dulcie might say "great minds", I'd say "convergent evolution of thought" – both of us would say: "There is nothing (nowt) new under the sun". We'd just like to acknowledge some of our kindred thinkers, speakers and providers who we have only recently discovered online as we have come to complete converting The52Tips blogs into this book:

• The Marshall Skills Academy:

www.cambridgenetwork.co.uk/news/get-your-daily-dose-happiness

• Mind My Peelings:

www.mindmypeelings.com/blog/daily-dose-of-happiness-chemicals

- Kaia Roman, author of The Joy Plan:
www.mindbodygreen.com/articles/trigger-happy-chemicals
- Nicole Lazzaro on Clark Bucker's B2B Nation's technology Advice podcast:
https://technologyadvice.com/blog/information-technology/
activate-chemicals-gamify-happiness-nicole-lazzaro/
- Wellington Multiple Sclerosis (supporting people with MS)
https://mswellington.org.nz/wp-content/uploads/2021/11/
Your-Daily-Green-DOSE-V1.pdf

If you have also 'found' / 'thought out' DOSE as a model for yourself, or found it elsewhere, do connect with us – we'd love to see this as a model that can help as many as possible together.

Secondly, to paraphrase the great British statistician and thinker George Box: 'all models are fallible, some are useful'. The amazing and enormous complexity of the brain's biology means that such chemicals (neurotransmitters and hormones) are only some of the ones in play, and each has very specific local actions (sometimes counterintuitively so), as well as more global brain or body ones too. This is also before we even consider the multitude of chemical receptors and their different functions. To be healthy, some chemicals require balancing rather than an ever-long pursuit of more i.e., more is not always better. So, as a self-pharmaceutical-styled model, DOSE can only ever be part of the 'answer'. To really help ourselves and others to greater happiness requires the concurrent and strategic neural 'rewiring', and 'maintenance' of that wiring, that occurs by doing such #Tips, consistently and stacking them. This is the real 'power' of the approach and what we are advocating in The52Project and this book.

Acknowledgements

There are so many people to thank when you have an idea that rather wonderfully turns into a project.

For the process of this project 'becoming', we are indebted to so many for their generous and ongoing inspiration, support and encouragement for this project and book and in making it a reality. At its heart The52Project and @the52tips was, and is, an ongoing community project. We believe in our friend and colleague's Andrew Jenkins' maxim for LeadersLiveTV "I to the power of we".

To all those that joined, or watched back or gave feedback on, our weekly Friday morning Instagram Lives in 2021, thank you!

We would like to say a special BIG THANK YOU to our live guests and contributors:

Firstly, to Jen (AKA DigitalJen / Jen Smith), for creating the fastest website in the west ever, and for formulating so many #Tips with and for us, for being our most committed tester (experimenter), supporter, critical friend, regular co-presenter / guest and all-round web, blog and tech guru. This project, this book, would not exist without you. Jen you are one of the best!

Tip Contributors

Cathy Hart (#Tip**5** 'And Breathe' & #Tip**18** 'Sing it Out')
@cathyhartvocals / @cathyhartcoaching / www.cathyhart.co.uk

Hedge Haigh (#Tip**6** 'Do the Plank' & #Tip**20** 'Roll With it')
@hedgehaighpt / www.warwickpersonaltrainer.com

Hannah Powell (#Tip**11** 'Small Moments Matter')
@thecactussurgeon / www.thecactussurgeon.com

Amy Leighton (#Tip**16** 'Brew and Dance' and stand in co-presenter for #Tip**31** 'Let it Go' & #Tip**33** 'Cut it Out')
@amyleighton 6/ www.amyleighton.com

Jen Smith (#Tip**12** 'Playlist for Life', #Tip**17** 'Colour Matters', #Tip**22** 'Flip it', #Tip**26** 'Ripple Effect', #Tip**30** 'Make Something of it', #Tip**34** 'Find Your Flock', #Tip**36** 'Managing Monsters', #Tip**37** 'Wait for it', #Tip**43** 'Fright it', #Tip**48** 'Slow it Down', #Tip**49** 'Joy of Missing Out (JOMO)', #Tip**51** 'Offer it', #Tip**52** 'Pass it On')
@digi_jen / www.digitaljen.co.uk

Nikki Yeomans (#Tip**19** 'Blink or You'll Miss it')
@i.fix.me / www.ifixme.co.uk

Helen Guinness (#Tip**23** 'Time to Reframe it')
@guinness.helen / https://helenguinness.com

James Bushe (#Tip**24** 'Sleeping in Sync')
@bushepilot / www.jamesbushe.com

Kimberley Owen (#Tip**25** 'Game on!')
@craftbeerpinup / @hellokimberleyo / @tedxleam

Jen Rolfe (#Tip**26** 'Ripple Effect')
@not_just_a_princess / www.practicallypositive.com

Caroline Laycock (#Tip**27** 'The One Thing')
https://getmoredoneatwork.com / www.linkedin.com/in/caroline-laycock-34259132

Dave Rogers (#Tip**28** 'Mood Hoovers')
@fuelledfitandfiredup / https://fuelledfitandfiredup.com

Katie Maycock (#Tip**29** 'Breakfast Brain')
@getyourshittogether.io / www.getyourshittogether.io

Mike Taylor (#Tip**31** 'Let it Go')
@mike.a.taylor / https://youtu.be/asJA6HDzkWk (ShedTV)

Joe Rowntree (#Tip**41** 'The Best Medicine')
@joe.rowntreecomedian / www.joerowntree.com

Louise Sugden (#Tip**43** 'Fright it')
@loulousuggers / https://louisesugden.co.uk

Dr Afiniki Akanet (#Tip44 'Keep it')
@aakanet / www.afiniki.co.uk

Leigh Laramy (#Tip48 'Slow it Down')
https://www.linkedin.com/in/leigh-laramy-849a58105/

Sara Sibai (#Tip50 'Play')
@sarasibai / www.inplayfulcompany.com

To photographer extraordinaire Darren Robinson, we marvel at your craft of lighting and subject angles (#Tip22) and framing (#Tip23).

Editors Karen Tomlinson Burling and David Hambling thank you so much for all your time and efforts in taking our www.The52Project.com blogs and wrestling them into manageable drafts and then subsequent drafts into the final polished articles. We know crafting us into fewer words is a huge challenge!

Sarah Walden of Noodle Juice Ltd, for producing this book: for your endless patience, efficiency, wisdom, cajoling, discipline, incentivising, 'red pen' and most of all belief in making The52Project / @the52tips accessible as a book.

Thanks to Helen Hambleton, Zoe Gallimore and Lucy Funnell at People Untapped for bringing us into your PU family, introducing us to each other and lending your support, time and energy behind the scenes at many different points - personal and professional.

Thanks to Jamie Swanston for the 'The52Project' title – created that same first Saturday night!

Thanks to Kimberley Owen and Amy Leighton for your patience in introducing us to Instagram Lives and your early faith that we'd each be good on the very small screen.

Seriously you would not be reading this if Dulcie had never met Sarah, Karen and Jen and then introduced Iain. We talk about Find Your Flock (#Tip34) and these are among our immediate work tribe who have a hand in almost everything we do when it looks good and sounds professional. They are some of our favourite people to drink a cuppa, or wine or eat cake with too, so that's something to put on the gratitude list (#Tip3) on its own.

To our charity partner The Big Issue Foundation (www.bigissue.com/big-issue-foundation) – thank you for all that you do for so many and being an inspiration for community projects for us all.

A very special thank you to all the lovely early followers that kept us going with their encouraging feedback and regularly turning up to say hello on Fridays' Instagram Lives at 10am (UK time) in 2021! Many of you turned into the guests above. To those not already mentioned above, we're sending an extra special 'wave' to some of our early regulars Helen Melvin, Jane Althorpe, Nikki Blackhurst, Sarah Walden,

David Brambell, John Lambert, Anna Price, Linda Stephens, Moira Shepherd, Pops, Emma (Emmi-lou), Auntie Rita, Annelise Swanston, Tamarah Khatib, Helen Stuttard, Matt Howcroft, Rachel Burgess, Oana Gherasim, and Amelie Cobb. Together with our guests you made the crucible from which this project started to really take shape and 'become'.

We would also like to thank our eagle-eyed early readers; Caroline Laycock, Lisa Price, Helen Melvin, Cass Coulston, Karen Tomlinson Burling, Graham Kirk, Zoe Gaffney and Matthew Howcroft, who all took time out of their busy pre-Christmas schedules to spot typos, the odd grammatical error and, in one instance, a missing chapter! Don't worry, we found it and it's back in!

Finally, and most importantly, for the ongoing tireless support and forbearance of our respective families. THANK YOU for your ongoing love and patience as we both prepared, tried out, wrote, endlessly edited and talked about these #Tips. Thank you also for often being our smartphone camera operators! Lastly, thank you so much for allowing us to be the embarrassing triggers for science and well-being that we are.

References

There are many references for the science included in this book so we thought, rather than increasing the length of the book and using up more paper, we would embrace technology and let you find them online.

So if you are interested in reading more about the science we have discussed in each #Tip, either head over to:

https://the52project.com/references/

Or scan the whizzy QR code below and it will take you to the same place.